POSITIVELY
TAROT

POSITIVELY TAROT

A Modern Guide to
A Mindful Life

EMMA
TOYNBEE

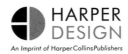

HARPER
DESIGN
An Imprint of HarperCollins Publishers

To my divinely driven mum, whose ever-present,
affirmatory and expansive approach subsequently
shaped the life of her firstborn grandchild:
cradled close and speaking their first words
in our tending reader's hands

First published in the UK in 2018 by Thorsons,
an imprint of HarperCollins Publishers

Positively Tarot.

HarperCollins books may be purchased for educational,
business, or sales promotional use. For information
please email the Special Markets Department
at SPsales@harpercollins.com.

Published in 2019 by

Harper Design

An Imprint of HarperCollins*Publishers*
195 Broadway
New York, NY 10007
Tel: (212) 207-7000
Fax: (855) 746-6023
harperdesign@harpercollins.com
www.hc.com

Distributed throughout North America by
HarperCollins*Publishers*
195 Broadway
New York, NY 10007

ISBN 978-0-06-289938-5

Library of Congress Control Number 2018963507

Printed in China
First Printing, 2019

WHY THIS BOOK?

The tarot has traditionally been used as an esoteric tool for divination purposes, but in the modern day it can be so much more. Anyone and everyone can benefit from reading the tarot, from business professionals to stay-at-home parents. We all need help from time to time to navigate the ups and downs of life, whether it comes from friends, partners, family, teachers, therapists, counsellors, life coaches, preachers or a guru. But no matter to whom we look for higher wisdom and guidance, rarely can they match the complete honesty and instant availability of the tarot. A session with a professional life coach or therapist can be invaluable at any time in life, whether we are in a crisis or simply needing some regular time dedicated to our own personal evolution and development. Yet that session can't always be perfectly aligned with our impulse to seek out reassurance. The tarot is available day and night, at whatever time and place is most convenient for us to absorb its lessons; all we have to be is ready and willing to improve the quality of our thoughts, and subsequently our life.

Tarot pushes the black-hole button in the brain. It prompts the rational mind to relinquish control and instantly grant access to previously inaccessible information – and knowledge empowers. In life and business, the tarot can be a go-to device, taking our mind to places it never would otherwise have entered and enabling us to crack any impedimental imbalances or stalemates and move forward. Tarot is about seeing meaning and connections and finding purpose, but also, now more than ever, reworking the mind so that it functions naturally, organically and healthily. We now know what the information age looks and feels like and are starting to realize the impact the rapid advance of technology can have on our personal lives, business and society. The rapid processing power of computerized devices is becoming a substitute for our own judgement, intuition and deeper understanding through direct experience. In short, the computerized world has many benefits, but has also become a kind of mind-crutch, allowing the cognitive brain to call less and less on the limbic intuitive centre.

One of the effects of the ubiquitous information overload is a sort of analytical paralysis; the sheer amount of information available to us is so overwhelming that we tend to give up the chase and select only the information that confirms a pre-existing condition or belief. It's time to rise up and reclaim the brain. Rather than being pigeonholed by our usual 'online' preferences, we will find that tarot gives our mind a chance to completely refresh itself and avoid getting stuck in automated algorithmic thought ruts.

Tarot is the point when art and science meet, where we can see the workings of the subconscious mind in material reality. I believe that the most profound and modern application of the tarot is as an inner emotional or psychological mind map, showing where and how our current frame of mind is driving our life. When following any map, as we know, even the smallest degree of adjustment to our planned trajectory can take us miles off-course. Using the tarot as a mind map, we are able to backtrack, fast-track and pinpoint how our behavioural responses, reactions or non-reactions can either lead us back to the start or down a new and exciting life path.

All becomes possible with the tarot deck as our mobile future tap, including predicting the outcome of a meeting, how a particularly tricky client, or the markets, will react, and whether a stock or project is worth a punt. We can also be poised and prepared when something is about to have its moment, and foresee financial, business or fashion trends – and so, in a sense, make them. The liquid modern world often requires an ultra-open and fluid response, and tarot reading helps generate new neural pathways and allows us to be continually reassessing and reinventing. In today's fast-moving and ever-changing world, in this era of quick-fixes and information, the tarot can keep us ahead of the ever-pacier game.

In addition to its honest and transparent approach to problem-solving, when used as a form of pocket guru, wisdom teacher or counsellor, the tarot can help reclaim our misplaced power. We can misplace our power by becoming too reliant on others for our own psycho-emotional care or support. They then become like props or crutches, and we are not given the opportunity to grow and mature through our own self-reliance. Using the tarot as a psycho-emotional map offers us a way of reclaiming any unnecessary drains on our personal power, leading to ever-greater self-esteem and emotional security.

When we are stuck, facing a problem or lacking perspective, the symbolic imagery of the tarot can also stimulate our latent intuition, allowing us to overcome the obstacle of ignorance and reorient ourselves in a positive and constructive direction. Tarot can be used in any unclear situation when there's a decision to be made or problem to be solved: no valley is too deep and no mountain too high for the divinely inspired. Yet, paradoxically, we need not climb, jump, leap or even fly to the highest ground, for the teleporting tarot-freed mind, which recognizes no such material limitations, can take us there instantaneously. Pure intuition – those anomalous thoughts that drop in from nowhere – are the lateral mind's innate way of avoiding the queue of slower-moving logical, rational and reasoning lines of thought. Intuition relies on the fastest part of the brain – the limbic system

– and is considered to be 80,000 times faster than our cognitive thought processes. The limbic system quickly and easily communicates feelings and bits of information to our conscious intelligence to maximize our chances of survival in a threatening context. Artists know how to access and use their intuition, but they need many years of studio practice to hone it. For those who don't have the time or inclination for artistic practices, the tarot offers another 'in-house' mind-tapping option. So this book is, in a sense, simply a user's guide to the mind, to help access as yet untapped aspects of intuitive brain functioning.

The tarot also provides a sacred space in which we can examine and observe the phenomena that arise or are constructed in our mind. Many ancient and modern minds agree, be they teachers, preachers, scientists, philosophers, heads of state or business moguls, that our thoughts create our reality. So, by knowing ourselves and the inner workings of our own mind, we can make the very best of life and positively augment our reality.

For me, the most exciting, relevant and contemporary use of the tarot is as a psychological tool to render us more effective, balanced and constructive individuals in our own lives and society. Most tarot books give an explanation of what's happening on the outside, but rarely do they answer this all-important 'Why me?' question. So these books, like a quick-fix doctor offering curative but not preventative treatments, are the sort that will keep seeing their readers again and again, always with the same complaint. By identifying our own psychology or life philosophy as the root cause of our external life experience, however, we are able to effect lasting change. So, rather than write another quick-fix tarot book, I decided to take a more holistic and preventative approach, to serve my readers' prospects better in the long term.

By proper use of the tarot for the purpose of deeper self-reflective enquiry, we can thoroughly examine and judge our words, deeds and actions, and weigh their consequences. This process teaches us to pay more attention, to know our uncultivated selves better, to look inwardly in order to successfully enrich our outer lives. In so doing, we can also recognize and appreciate the moral and noble qualities of our spirit and character, as well as those qualities that aren't serving us and need to be transcended. In seeing ourselves clearly, we are able to draw back the veil that conceals our destiny.

The tarot also helps us process the conflict we as humans face in the duality of our personal impulses – the material, physical body drawn towards sensual pleasure and the ethereal higher-dimensional body drawn towards the elevated mind and spirit. The tarot helps us recover our truest, purest, most shining expression of being, so we can finally attain the perfect sense of our spirit belonging, or at-one-ment in our physical body. There really is no greater gift we can give ourselves than the use of this ultimate self-realization tool, for, like those who love us, the divinely inspired tarot wants only the very best for us.

With so many possibilities, it is not surprising that in all the years I have been reading and teaching tarot card reading, the one question I am asked again and again by clients and students is: 'How do you know which interpretation to choose?' When you look at the various tarot books available, each gives a myriad of options for interpretation, but none a system of how to navigate the labyrinth of possibilities and get transparent, straightforward answers. So this is also a book that addresses this issue.

I have found the reading of tarot cards becomes inefficient when we focus too much on the individual elements of each card. Fragmenting the images in this way only serves to slow our mental processing of the cards' bigger picture; intuition works twice as quickly as logical analysis, so I have created a book that doesn't spend pages breaking down the images into their component parts, but synthesizes the information to provide conclusive, resolved and up-to-date statements. When learning tarot, I found clarity, quick referencing and go-to statements far more useful than reams of outdated and impedimental image analysis. Remembering that the figure in the Eight of Cups wears a red cape to denote action, when half the cards in the deck denote some form of action, did not serve to increase my proficiency as a tarot reader. In this book I haven't shunned symbol analysis completely, but I've used it sparingly, and only if relevant or accessible to modern-day conditions.

This is a book for beginners, improvers and those looking to add a level of professionalism to their readings. It works for those who are right-brain dominated, relying on instinct and intuition, and those who are left-brain dominated, with strong logical and reasoning abilities. With the aid of this book you don't need to be the all-seeing eye to give a profound, accurate and discerning card reading. Jump from amateur straight to professional standard – this fast-track guide will take you quickly and efficiently to the highest level of competence in your tarot readings.

PART I

TAROT
INTERPRETATION

THE POWER OF SYMBOLS
AND IMAGERY

The tarot is a centuries-old tradition that relies on the power of imagery. We tend to remember images better than concepts; we see images around us and our brain responds. The visual aspect of movies, television, picture books and magazines speaks to us on a deep level that doesn't require the explanation of words alone. The images of the tarot are particularly powerful, being made up of symbols rooted in ancient traditions. The information they carry is deeply embedded in our subconscious mind without us even cognitively realizing it, making the tarot a particularly powerful set of images. Through its triggering of specific unconscious responses, it stretches our cognitive legs, and thus, via this divinely heightened and wider-striding perspective, we can leap all cognitive mind hurdles to access whatever information is needed. The answer to any question is always there, buried in our own mind.

Putting Ourselves in the Picture

A common question people often ask themselves during a difficult, challenging or crisis situation is 'Why me?' Knowing the answer to this question can be invaluable to getting ahead and leading a life filled with triumphs, successes and abundance.

To know the exact role our mental processes are playing in our situation is of paramount importance. Our frame of mind can be fertile and expansive, ready to make the best of any new opportunity, or sterile and inhibitive, holding us back from enjoying a fuller and happier life. Which mode of operating is in charge at any given time doesn't have to be hidden in the deepest recesses of our mind. By using the tarot as a psychological magnifying glass, we can bring a fuller conscious awareness to any inhibiting mental processes and in so doing lift their restrictions and limitations on our life experience.

Tweaking the inner workings of our mind can then help us avoid destructive or toxic fictional narratives. For instance, by addressing any tendencies towards denial, scarcity or poverty, our consciousness can enable us to allow ourselves the experiences of love, wealth, health or fulfilment in our work.

The unrefined mind is like a roughly hewn lump of stone or masonry, which makes for an ineffective building material. To create a balanced, stable block that we can effectively and constructively use for building, we need to work the stone, to chip away at it, to keep perfecting, refining and flattening its rough edges. Only when it is perfectly flat and smooth, devoid of any bumps, lumps and imperfections, will it be ready for use in building a stable structure, a structure that will stand the tests of a lifetime.

The idea that what we put into life we get out can be seen very clearly when we start this process of chipping away at our own mind; for every lump and bump smoothed over in our mind, an equal and opposite reaction occurs in our external environment, so paths and impediments clear and the rocky roads of life become that little bit smoother and more negotiable.

The more we work with the tarot in this way, by viewing our own psychology as the main building contractor for our reality, the more stable our world becomes. Where, on the other hand, there is little awareness or scrutiny of our own psychological construction methods, they become nightmare cowboy builders, destabilizing and eternally patching up the building of our life.

The idea that the inner workings of our own mind should remain largely elusive and enigmatic seems strangely inconsistent with the open-access ideal of the information era. As the world around us becomes increasingly optimized and efficient via computerization and robotics, the mind becomes the optimal nut to crack. Impervious to such updates, it often presents the greatest challenge of them all.

If we allow it to be, the tarot can be our own private and personal detective, uncovering the workings of our own mind. Using this system, we can objectively observe the dialogue between the higher, enquiring and equality-seeking aspect of our mind and the domineering ego aspect that usually prefers to remain anonymous, for to be recognized and labelled would imply that we had conscious awareness of its otherwise hidden power over us. But *Positively Tarot* is all about putting ourselves back in the picture: looking at our life with a greater sense of the part we have to play in moulding and shaping it. Rather than being a bystander, passively observing while our ego mind takes us on an unnecessarily bumpy ride, we can awaken and play a more active role creating our life.

If we allow the tarot to honour and serve our higher good by using it to forge a deeper and more honest relationship with ourselves, we will find that we reap the greatest and most profound of its benefits. For the finest thing we can ever offer ourselves is complete truth and honesty; it is only from that stabilized point that we can build a life full of greater meaning, purpose and fulfilment. When our mind begins to focus on transparency and honesty, starting with itself, the rest of our world also comes into a clearer, sharper focus, and this is the magical key to physical and material manifestation.

The more awareness we direct to the fact that our thoughts create our reality, the more control we can take back. When we shuffle the tarot cards and lay out a spread, it will always show what narrative role our own mind is playing in a situation, and how and what it is creating, allowing or attracting. For the tarot works on a 'like attracts like' basis, mirroring the workings of our own mind in our external environment.

Cognition versus Intuition

Most people, especially in business, rely wholly on the cognitive part of the brain – the neocortex – to evaluate key or critical situations before they choose how best to proceed. It's what our modern education system encourages as part of our formative training, and thus, once the foundations are set, like a wind-up automaton, it is often difficult to break or override these behavioural patterns. When decision-making on a day-to-day basis, we can slip into a somnambulist state, sleepwalking through life, following the same pre-programmed coding and producing adequate but not particularly original or transformative results.

The growing epidemic of the 'automaton mind' is reflected in our external consensus reality via our increasing reliance on automation robotics, Excel spreadsheets, Data Science and Business Intelligence. While these are powerful tools, they render the internal and inextricable external landscape flat, devoid of the beautifully orchestrated learning curves, the creative glitches and errors fundamental to the way we naturally learn and from which our most unique, original, innovative and inventive thought processes are derived. In the automated landscape there is no room for error, no room for chaos, or for the type of mistakes that give rise to opportunity.

There is a deep irony to what is done in the name of progress having the equal and opposite consensus reaction in the human psyche, and bringing our higher development, due largely to emotional self-reliance, to a complete standstill. It seems now that a gradual refining or perfecting of the character, via myriad accidents, mistakes or errors of judgement, gives a crucial opportunity for the psyche to grow, change and transform, and this is becoming much delayed as we become more dependent on external processing machines and less on our own processing abilities.

The infantilizing devices upon which everyone so heavily relies are replacing the parental and grandparental wisdom that allows, via human fallibility, for us to make mistakes and learn from them. Young minds now profess to 'know' not through their own direct experience, but via online prophets' second-, third-, fourth- and fifth-hand inexperience. Suddenly individual subjectivity is being superseded by indirect objectivity: the antithesis of the magical principle that lies in each and every one of us – the freedom to directly experience the unseen. So the mind is moved ever closer to mundane concerns and levels of operating and away from the unfathomable divine and sacred aspect.

It is ironic that with the rise of all-pervasive modern technologies, the world as augmented by our own direct experience should have become so closed off and shallow. At the same rate as the world is seemingly opening up, the modern cult of mundane, sense-perceived, reductive reality is closing it off, packaging it neatly inside an egoistic, all-knowing box.

When a real-life decision is needed, the information-numbed, automatic data-crunching mind cannot provide a unique, original, radically innovative answer. Only the autonomous intuitive mind can make such leaps into the unknown, and there it waits, quietly ahead of forever-increasing lengths of cognitive 'real time', for the latter-day mind to catch up. Sometimes this can take days, or weeks, or months, or years, making this an inefficient and ineffective method of decision-making. Thus the seemingly progressive information era, in terms of human evolution and development, is as impedimental as a tightly plot-ted farce played by business moguls or politicians instead of trained actors, i.e. *sans* entertainment or comedy.

Fortunately, the quiet higher clarity or transparency of the intuitive mind has ways and means of making itself heard, both on- and offline. The tarot provides a platform, raising up this objectifying voice so that it might speak and be heard. When it is heard, and uncorrupted by lower, base or unwise motivations or instincts, we can wholly trust it. Both our own and others' intuitions or gut feelings can be relied on to resolve the trickiest problems or make even the most difficult decisions.

When several options seem equally attractive, perhaps due to too many unseen criteria, the tarot can also help us to make a clear and incisive choice. Making everyday decisions shouldn't be like fiction, where the mind seeks an entertaining, dramatic and diverting narrative route from A to B; the tarot avoids such unnecessary convolutions and takes us to where we want to be authentically, precisely, directly.

In more important decisions – when we, for example, meet a new love interest or a candidate for a job – our brain begins data-crunching, and decision-making can be delayed and pro-ress impeded due to the need for further information or analysis. The mind, the biggest data-collector in the world, can even remain stuck in a never-ending narrative. The tarot reminds us, by the very ritualistic practice of shuffling the cards, that linear thinking can be predictably circuitous and that it is intui-tive leaps that take us into new, exciting, unknown territory.

Whether a life or business decision is successful or not is often down to timing. The tarot is also ideal for showing us not just what and where, but most importantly when the time is right to move or act.

Unfortunately, intuitive or 'anomalous' thinking – seeing or creating a connection between seemingly unrelated concepts – is

THE POWER OF SYMBOLS AND IMAGERY

too often disregarded by the conscious cerebral cortex as irrational and nonsensical. When intuition gives the answer at faster-than-light speed, the analytical overlay of the logical mind tries, and often fails, to make sense of it: a series of error messages flashes on our mind screen, making it impossible to progress until we override the errors by finding something physical or external to clear or clarify the intuitive position. Of course, this often doesn't happen, at least not immediately, so the intuitive information is unconsciously trashed.

The more conscious attention and awareness we give to our mental dynamics, i.e. intuition versus cognition, however, the more we will begin to notice the error messages, and when we catch them in time we can choose to cancel and accept them, rather than allow the unconscious mind to continually trash its greatest resource.

This is how all tarot players are winners: by allowing themselves the time and opportunity to consciously question the validity and authority of their own subtle internal messaging system and then to take advantage of it.

Eventually, as our faith in our mind's intuitive response becomes stronger, the error messages will become less frequent and less insistent. After using the tarot for some months, we will notice, when observing our mind's response, how the cognitive dialogue has changed from being bold, capitalized and domineering to medium, lower-case and quiet, even sheepish, following the intuitive dialogue rather than leading our mind, and indeed life, in a not very merry dance.

Intuition, the Next Intelligence

The founder and CEO of Amazon, Jeff Bezos, observed that 'There are decisions that can be made by analysis. These are the best kind of decisions. They are fact-based decisions that overrule the hierarchy. Unfortunately, there's this whole other set of decisions you can't boil down to a math problem.' What he was alluding to was, arguably, the hallmark of Amazon's success: its capacity to make big decisions based on intuitive hunches.

Some people do retain their competitive positions by utilizing fact-based information and knowledge more effectively than others. But with information now ubiquitous, unregulated and freely accessible via the internet, traditional sources of advantage must dig even deeper. Thus the most successful individuals in the future will be likely to be dualistically smart in their information sourcing, harnessing other innate tools in combination with conditioned responses, pure logic and rational analysis. That is to say, harnessing their lightning-flashes of intuition.

As the fastest, smartest, most reliable and trustworthy aspect of brain functioning, intuition can remove any blocks and get the river running freely and easily once again. With its ability to transform any sphere of human existence, it has to be the next step in human intelligence. And just as the ancient Chinese philosopher Sun Tzu's treatise of military strategy *The Art of War* is now considered a business classic, so the ancient and equally versatile tradition of tarot card reading, with its unlimited applications, will come to the fore, I believe, as a way of accessing latent intuition.

Windows of Transparency

Symbolic imagery, as noted earlier, is a way of accessing uncharted territories of the mind. Science says we only use 10 per cent of our brain, suggesting if we can only reach them, the unexploited resources of the mind are in plentiful supply. The imagery of the tarot opens the way to them. It is fantastical and of another era. It evokes a sense of the unknown, that which isn't learned or conditioned and can't be taught, but can be as individual as we are.

The key principle of the tarot adheres to the Zen Buddhist concept of the Buddha Mind being a beginner's mind, meaning to know, or to think so, is to close our mind to other possibilities. The superior form of knowing is not to know, which sounds almost Wonderlandesque, but, as Lewis Carroll, and the proverbial 'mad' scientist, well understood, there is method in the nonsensical 'madness' of the unconscious. The tarot's arcane and ambiguous visual hooks keep the intuitive and clarity-carving centres of the brain engaged and, like Alice, ever wondering.

To understand the tarot imagery correctly we must analyse it in the same way that a psychotherapist or psychologist would a dream, with every symbolic element of each card being understood as a subconsciously operating aspect of our own psyche. Just as a dream provides pure, unadulterated information in a subtle symbolic and guiding form, the tarot can be equally penetrating, if we are pure and honest with ourselves.

For instance, when we look at a card like the Seven of Swords, which denotes a lone man walking away from his camp carrying more than just his own swords, what connotations does this have for us? What does our mind take from this scene? We can say that the man looks surreptitious, shady, dishonest, covert, hidden, undercover, clandestine, stealthy, veiled in his actions.

By applying this to our own psychology, we can understand how our own unconscious psycho-emotional mind works against itself, keeping itself in the dark and operating behind the scenes or remaining hidden from the attention of our own conscious awareness.

Swords denote thoughts, concepts and ideas, so, as the man is depicted carrying the swords of others, this card also shows that he is psychologically carrying the ideas and thoughts of others, which are creating his own self-concept, and a heavy self-concept at that, a concept that works against the idea of en-lightenment, healing and free movement. By carrying around others' ideas, our figure, an aspect of our own mind, is weighed down and his journey in life impeded.

It's a fine and privileged day indeed when we can finally rely solely on our own pure, higher-minded thoughts and en-lighten ourselves of the psycho-emotional load we carry, derived from others and supported by our own imaginative mind.

Tarot images are like windows of transparency, illuminating a thousand possible outcomes rather than just the narrow path of ignorance and shadow. They open and build new neural pathways, rather than closing them down via final or absolute words and statements. In this information age, intuitively freed thinking is the proverbial Sword of Truth, cutting through and revealing the stratification of linear thoughts in the over- or underbaked mind, life and the world as microcosms of the wider macrocosmic cake.

The tarot images are evocative, but not prescriptive. In fact they help the mind overcome such entrenched thinking, which is why the interpretive suggestions in this book should be taken as starting points and adapted to your own situation and style of card reading. Let's look now at how that can be developed.

TAROT READING

When laying out cards in the particular, traditional order of tarot reading, we go through a ritual, a necessary Zen-like process that calms our analytical and automatized data-crunching mind. Meditatively shuffling, laying and turning the cards helps us to switch off the calculating-ego aspect of the mind and re-engage with an omniscient or at-one-mentality.

The handling, shuffling, laying out and reading of tarot cards provides a precious few moments of personal, private time, without the online world of commerce watching. When the shuffled and selected cards appear in specific positions, each having a particular meaning in itself but also in relation to the other cards present, the linear narrative of the tarot, which speaks to our logical, rational cognitive processes, is reordered, and the symbolic imagery begins speaking, subtly and indirectly, in the language of the subconscious. When addressed in its own language, the subconscious is then free to speak back – to enter into a dialogue with the archetypal figures depicted in the cards. Hence the tarot system is a key to unlocking the deepest part of the inner self as well as providing answers to both sacred and mundane questions.

Divination or Self-Realization?

This book is written to honour the higher function of the tarot, as a tool for greater self-awareness and realization, understanding that the powers of divination and future prediction are but by-products of this deeper process of psychic purification and refinement. Allowing yourself to be driven by the motive of attaining extra-sensory perceptive powers will have the opposite effect: like a fly caught in a spider's web, the more forcibly the ego strives and struggles to get ahead, the more stuck or fixed your position in life becomes.

So the first and most crucial stage in seeking intuitive-level clarity is to unclutter your mind of any convoluted ego projections, motivations and agendas. Forging a completely honest, transparent, self-realized relationship with yourself is the only way to ensure you are a pure channel and giving absolutely accurate readings, whatever your purpose.

Reading the Cards: A Quick-Start Guide

- When sitting down to read the cards, you should find a quiet space where you are unlikely to be interrupted.
- You must then decide whether you want to do a general life reading, look only at a specific area of life or find an answer to a specific question.
- Then, looking in the layouts section at the back of the book (*page 313*), select a layout that you feel will provide the most interesting and relevant reading or answer to your question.
- Now, taking the entire deck, shuffle the cards in whichever way you find most comfortable, making sure you keep the cards image side down so you see only the generic backs of the cards.

Bear in mind, if you are reading the cards for someone else, that it is always the person asking the question and receiving the reading who must do the shuffling.

- While shuffling, hold the question you want answered in your mind, be it general or specific, until you intuitively feel the cards are sufficiently shuffled and ready to be laid down.
- Place the shuffled deck on the table in front of you (it's best to find a flat surface large enough to accommodate the number of cards shown in your chosen layout).
- Still holding your question or intention in mind, split the shuffled cards into three separate piles and, remembering the order in which you cut them, place them image side down. The piles don't have to be made equal, but can be if that is your preference.
- Then put the deck back together in a different way from how you split it.
- Now the cards are ready to be laid, image side down, in whatever layout you have chosen.
- To lay the cards, first choose a number between one and seven, or, if you are reading for someone else, ask them to choose this number.
- Say the number you choose is seven, first remove six cards from the top of the deck and place them to one side, so it is the seventh card that you place in position one of your chosen layout. Then, to lay the second card in the layout, do the same again, removing another six cards from the top of the deck, so it is the seventh card that you place in position two of the reading. Keep discarding six cards and laying only the seventh card until every card in the layout has been placed.
- Once the cards are in position, you can begin to turn them over, so the image side faces up and is the right way round. You can either turn all the cards over at once, or, if you are new to tarot reading, it may be more beneficial to follow the sequential order

specified for your chosen layout and turn the cards over one at a time. If you are a beginner, turning the cards slowly and individually will help you to fully absorb the lessons contained within each card before seeing how the story unfolds by moving on to the next. It is easy for beginners to become overwhelmed and despondent when faced with the large amount of information present in a multiple card reading, hence it is best for those new to tarot reading to take the step-by-step approach rather than trying to read the cards as a synthesized whole.

Using the intuitive go-to statements provided in this book as a starting point, you can now start to piece together a narrative framework in relation to your posed question or area of interest. On each of the cards pages that follow you will find words and ideas that will form a gateway between your conscious and subconscious. Basic key phrases for each card are **emboldened for the purposes of quicker referencing** to help refresh the memory of those who are familiar with the tarot and to help new users to grasp the basic meaning of each card.

While analysing each card individually is the necessary first step in learning to read the tarot, the tone a specific card has, rather than the basic symbolic ideas it presents, can shift depending on the type of influence specific to the others surrounding it. Herein lies the art of reading tarot: *reading the cards together as a synthesized whole*, which is akin to viewing each card combination through a prism to assess any tonal variations, enhancements and augmentations of their basic textbook definitions. This is what I hope the connective structuring of book will help you achieve, via its synthesized and bracketed suggestions of how various card combinations can play out.

Bear in mind that the ideas on these pages that inexplicably resonate or provoke an uncomfortable, rather than flattering, gratifying, indulging or obliging emotional reaction, are those with the potential, if the guidance is integrated, to induce the greatest growth, change and transformation.

Major and Minor Arcana

The tarot deck consists of seventy-eight cards: twenty-two Major Arcana cards, ranging from the Fool as card o to the World as card 22, and fifty-six Minor Arcana cards.

Each of the Major Arcana cards, which represent the major forces and events at work in the situation, depicts an archetypal character or scene, as you might find when analysing the individual driving forces in a fictional tale. Each archetype is distinctly different, embodying a uniquely individual type of psychology, philosophy, spirituality or pattern of behavioural response. Archetypes might have diametrically different responses to exactly the same personal or professional life situation. For example, though the Devil and the High Priestess both deal in hidden matters, the latter is morally and ethically grounded in their words and actions, whereas the former is not.

The fifty-six Minor Arcana cards are divided into four suits: Wands, Cups, Pentacles and Swords. They depict the minor events that occur as a result of the Major Arcana's life-force archetypes.

Just as the knocking over of the first domino in a line will knock down the rest, so the Major Arcana cards set off a chain reaction to produce the situations and events depicted in the Minor Arcana. Therefore I have extended the twenty-two Major Arcana card sections to incorporate a deeper study and analysis of which key human interest areas will trigger a particular response from each unique archetype. These sections are broken down as follows: personification and psychology; spirituality and philosophy; personal life; professional life; property, finances and resources; health and well-being.

The four suits of the Minor Arcana need no such breaking down, as each, by design, deals specifically with one of the four key areas of human concern: the Wands, physical energy and action; the Cups, feelings and emotions; the Pentacles, money and material acquisitions; the Swords, thought processes and intellect.

Advancing your Tarot Reading

As the English poet and cleric John Donne said in 1624, 'No man is an island,' and by finding similar themes and symbolism repeated throughout the cards, you can begin to form a mental web or network of connections between the different narrative themes, scenes and characters of the Major and Minor Arcana. For instance, the symbols of the upright sword, Sun/daylight and Moon/night are featured many times throughout the deck, so in grasping the meaning of these symbols and seeing and forming connections between the cards, you can begin to understand how the cards, when read in combination, work together as a whole.

For the advanced practitioner, who already has a good understanding of the meanings for the individual cards, I have placed abbreviations for all seventy-eight cards, embedded within brackets, throughout the card interpretation sections. These can be used to assist the reader in realizing the links between the cards and understanding how it is possible to quickly produce refined, succinct and wholly synthesized interpretations from the huge amount of raw symbolic information contained within a set of cards.

SUITS KEY CODE

W: Wands
C: Cups
P: Pentacles
S: Swords

An example of a key coded suit:

1C: Ace of Cups
2C: Two of Cups
3C: Three of Cups

and so on until the . . .

PC: Page of Cups
KnC: Knight of Cups
QC: Queen of Cups
KC: King of Cups

NB Only the suits are abbreviated; the Major Arcana card names appear in full.

Reading the Cards in Combination

While it is necessary for those who are new to tarot to first grasp the basic meanings of the cards, there will come a time when the beginner will hit a wall. Every tarot reader will reach this point, when they find that the simplistic style of reading the cards individually, without taking the relationship they have with any neighbouring cards into consideration, will no longer do. It is natural to want more depth and complexity from a tarot reading, for, after all, humans are complex creatures, made so by the dynamic tensions between the vital forces at play in their lives. This is where reading tarot cards in combination can become most useful and enlightening, by showing a fuller picture of all the influences, compulsions and impulses at work. Only by reading the cards in combination can we clearly see how the dynamic tensions and interplay between harmonious and inharmonious aspects of our psyche have a direct effect on our external reality and everyday life.

To really grasp the meaning of the cards in combination, it's important to remember that every card in the deck has its own unique relationship to each and every other, in the same sense that our energy, drives and impulses can be either compatible or incompatible with those of another individual. For example, by looking at the modus operandi of the Sun card, representing light, visibility, publicity, expression and autonomy, together with the regulatory reclusiveness of the Hermit or the conformist restrictions of the Hierophant, we can see how diametrically opposed are the overall 'game plans' of these archetypes. Thus, their combined energy in a reading will denote some significant and dynamic tension in our life.

Some archetypes are natural friends, others natural enemies. For example, the Sun surrounded by friendly, supportive or motivationally aligned cards, such as the King of Wands or Queen of Wands, with their naturally compatible outlook, can constructively empower our life and fuel great and positive growth, change and transformation.

When two oppositely motivated cards land next to each other in a reading, such as the Sun (purity, innocence, transparency) and the Devil (impurity, transgression, collusion), we can see how the latter can corrupt the former, creating the sort of difficulties and challenges that impede our growth and success in life.

When the cards placed next to each other in a reading have little or no relationship, being neutral or indifferent to one another, such as the Hermit and the Hierophant, this denotes a mixture of often lesser benefits but no impedimental difficulties, challenges or obstructions.

The key to understanding the role each card has to play in a synthesized multiple-card reading is remembering that the archetypal Major Arcana cards act as agents of, or lend agency to, their neighbouring cards. Taking the example below, you could read the combination of the High Priestess, the Sun, the World, the Eight of Wands and the Ace of Swords as: taking a contemporary, new look (1S: Ace of Swords) at an ancient spiritual system (High Priestess) of how to live a joyful and abundant life via self-realization (Sun) has led to the successful international (World) publication of this book (Sun), with the help of a quickly effective PR and marketing campaign (8W: Eight of Wands).

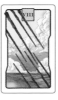

However the cards are combined, as aspects of our own psyche, it is of vital importance, if we wish to move forward quickly and easily with our plans, questions and life purpose, that any oppositely inclined internal forces are properly integrated and reconciled. Herein lies the beauty and power of the tarot, in providing the opportunity to make peace with the warring aspects of ourselves. After that, everything external falls perfectly into place.

PART II

TAROT CARDS

THE MAJOR ARCANA

The Major Arcana cards can set the tone for an entire reading. As the driving forces behind our impulses, thoughts, actions and general behaviour, they are by far the more interesting and complex of the two types of card. They indicate the root causes of all other minor life events, or indeed non-events, and are the lynch-pins around which all other events revolve. To understand these cards fully is to understand the general theme and schematics of our life. Most people look to the tarot when they want to make major changes or improvements to their lives, and to make such changes we must first address the underlying cause of the status quo, which is found only in the Major Arcana cards.

0 THE FOOL 0

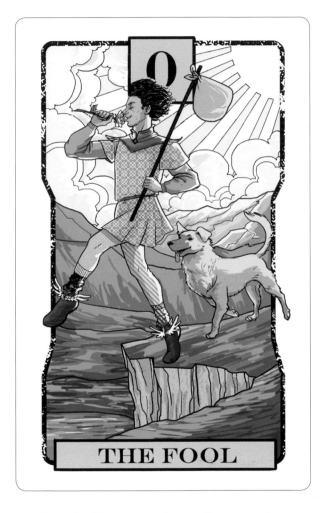

THE FOOL

'The only thing I know is that I know nothing.'
THE SOCRATIC PARADOX

Personification – Psychology

The archetypal Fool is a **carefree and fearless 'out-of-the-box' thinker (KS, QS, KnS) or activist (KW, QW, KnW)**, who exercises **complete and total liberality in everything they do**. Their **ever-open mind and freedom of spirit** make them interested in everyone and, usually, game for anything (World). They're a **flexible, spontaneous, go-with-the-flow type character**, whose life can, outwardly, appear **distinctly disorderly, detached and distanced**.

Those who embody the Fool archetype are often **inadvertently complacent, nonchalant, indifferent or apathetic (4C), distracted, unwitting, unsettled, scattered, thoughtless, mistaken or distracted in their behaviour. They often lose things** such as keys, wallet, phone, passport, jewellery, people, pets, track of time, etc.

Essentially, they are **a dreamer who lacks all forethought. Being blissfully (Sun) ignorant, oblivious, unaware of any potential risks or danger, they rarely look where they are going. Their complete lack of interest in what lies ahead and little or no concern for the future or the consequences of their actions (Judgement)** are both their best and worst character traits.

The Fool's **ultra-presence of mind can be seen in their mental disposition towards the short term**, which includes all forms of short-term arrangements and agreements or contracts (Justice). **Happy in the now**, they are unable to see what will bring satisfaction or emotional fulfilment in the long run (2S) – a long run off a short cliff.

They embody **a wilful and impulsive 'What have I got to lose?' mentality**. They are **the quintessential young idealist, whose unshaken belief or untested faith in their ideas** can seem both crazily naïve (Pages) to some and bravely innovative (Emperor) and creative (Empress) to others.

As **a pure, untainted, innocent and unsuspecting spirit,** the Fool can be **youthful and playfully childlike (6C) or childishly (Pages) self-absorbed (4P, 4C, 4S).** They are archetypically characterized by the Greek myth of Icarus, the son who precipitated his own death by ignoring his father's wise instruction and flying too close to the Sun. Whether the wax in the Fool's wings melts or not is much dependent on the surrounding and outcome cards.

The Fool's **ultra-present, happy-go-lucky state of mind** paradoxically underpins their dangerous inability to see beyond their own nose. **So weak are their personal boundaries (KC, QC, KnC, PC),** they can temporarily host another person's energy, be they a real, fictional or projected personality.

As a **pure, clean, blank, absorbent surface** upon which others can project their own wants, needs and desires (Moon), this archetype's **core self and personal preferences are often tucked beneath a blanket of external influences and persuasions.** Unless they learn to excavate this core self, perhaps via quiet contemplation or meditation (Hermit), they will find **the wilful ambitions of others can take advantage of their naturally apathetic nature (4C) and easily sway or influence them into making a series of inauthentic life choices (7C).**

Unless there are anti-Fool cards present (Hermit, Hierophant, High Priestess, Emperor) and acting as grounding agents to the Fool's **scattered behaviour,** this archetype, being prone to **the incoherent misappropriations of others' judgement, awareness, attention and even personality (Sun, 7S), will have trouble finding their true calling or vocation in life.**

Due to their weak boundaries, this archetype is prone to **saying or doing anything to keep the peace (Empress, Temperance),** often at the expense of their own needs (Moon), ethical code, morality (Hierophant), integrity (High Priestess, KS, QS) and even general sense of 'reality' (Moon, 7C).

The Fool also **obscures, obliterates, dissolves, disintegrates or blurs the boundaries and parameters** present in its neighbouring cards, be they physical, emotional, mental or spiritual; **the stronger another card's structure, order or belief system, the more the Fool-ish modus operandi will register as corrupting, trouble-making and contentious, despite the Fool having good intentions.**

This archetype often has **difficulty fathoming the socially correct response or reaction (Hierophant).** Their **indirect mode of confrontation, fearless ignorance and disconnection from, lack of interest in or total disregard (4C) for conventional social roles or conformist societal structures (Hierophant),** can, when left unchecked, eventually result in conflict (5W, 5S) and suffering, either their own or that of others (3S, 9S, 5C, 5C). However, when handled compassionately or sensitively (KC, QC, Strength, Temperance), some Fools manage **to find acceptable ways out of their otherwise encumbering social or cultural obligations.**

Spirituality and Philosophy

The appearance of the Fool in a reading can signify **a positive and effective phase of spiritual influence and enhancement,** often induced via **the total abandonment of material or sensual diversions and any falsely held hopes, ambitions or self-concepts.**

An ultra-present unburdening of the mind (Sun), induced via the Fool's **complete surrender to the here and now,** can confer ever greater healing and the dissolution of suffering (Star, Temperance).

By acting as an executive agent of the Divine, the **passive presence** of the Fool can crack our most encumbering psycho-emotional habits (Moon), the ones that block the healing and enlightenment process (Star).

The Fool's inadvertent philosophy on life is similar to that of the **Zen Buddhist concept of the beginner's mind: shedding, eradicating, relinquishing, distancing and detaching from all fixed knowledge and thought forms. The mutable mind of the Fool continually creates space for unlimited learning and understanding and a unified, uninterrupted connection with the all-knowing Divine (Magician, High Priestess).**

Combined with learned (Hierophant), wise, mature (Hermit), insightful (High Priestess), enlightening (Sun) or overseeing archetypes (World), the Fool embodies what is sometimes referred to as the Socratic paradox. However, when **under the sway of ignorant** or undeveloped influences (Pages, Knights), the Fool can project (Moon) a **foolhardy, emotionally unstable, ignorant, poorly informed or 'drink-talking' individual's dubious world view.**

Personal Life

In matters of relating to others, the Fool is **led by the heart and body, but not the head.** They often don't realize their **mistakes,** though innocently or inadvertently made, **in choosing a romantic partner** until things begin to fall apart (Tower, Death, 3S, 5C).

Being card zero in the deck, the Fool is concerned only with starting afresh (Aces) and **carries little or no emotional baggage from previous romantic involvements.**

This card either signifies **a detached and distanced relationship, the mutual relinquishing of emotional baggage (Judgement) or the undoing of negative emotional ego habits (Moon).**

Even when in a committed long-term relationship or marriage, the Fool-ish partner may seek various **extra-marital freedoms, without properly considering or caring about the consequences.**

Due to their **inherent detachment** and **unfixed tastes**, they usually don't have a 'type'. Instead, they are often **serial first-daters, seduced by the idea of love (7C), but turned off by the reality of it (4C).** They tend to **view all situations requiring a deeper involvement or commitment as wholly unsustainable,** and at that juncture will **quickly up and move on (KnW).**

Their signature move is the **innocent dissolution of emotional attachments (KnS, 1S, Emperor)**, whether they are outdated or not. Due to their **innocent, light-hearted, 'no-strings' romantic intentions (PC)**, what begins as a mere **dalliance or fling (Lovers)** can quickly and easily turn sour (3S, 5C, Tower, Death) when the Fool **fails to notice their lover's deepening emotional attachment.**

Due to their **unsettled and resolutely non-committal nature**, the Fool usually remains **emotionally uneducated, with an immature view of committed relationships (Pages).** Unless they wish to remain single, or celibate for spiritual purposes (Hermit, Hierophant), a possible solution to their **strong resistance to monogamy** is the forming of a **polygamous or open partnership (Lovers, 3W, 3C).**

Professional Life

In a combination reading with those archetypes still under development (Devil, Pages, Knights), the Fool is considered **uneducated, unknowledgeable, unwise, unaccomplished, ineffective and unworldly, with a great deal still to learn.** They often **peak too soon or finish too early, giving up when something needs more time to develop and mature.** When left unchecked, they can even be **detrimental to matters requiring solid grounding and great maturity of character.**

They often take jobs or enrol on courses with **little regard for their future trajectory. Remaining oblivious to the part they play** in precarious situations often leads to their **professional undo-ing**, resulting in job losses or business, project or exam failures (Death, Tower, 3S, 5P, 5C).

Their **career or study path is often continually interrupted**, like a bad phone signal. Their **enthusiastic starts** (Pages, Aces) often end abruptly when they discard, destroy or obliterate what they have accomplished. The Fool's signature move is trying to get ahead via **great, ill-considered leaps of faith** (Devil), which are often **badly misjudged**. Unqualified to meet the level of challenge, the overreaching Fool often falls flat on their face (Death).

Self-discipline, self-governance and direction are **great challenges** for Fools, as are following the rules of a management hierarchy (Emperor) or fitting into any form of organizational work structure (Hierophant). They are often the source of professional indiscretions, by ignoring or disrespecting **personal and professional boundaries**. For this reason, the Fool archetype frequently suffers through their **disconnection** from their work colleagues, or even their **abandonment** by those who would otherwise support their work or career (5C, 5P). Subsequently, theirs can be **a wandering, unsettled professional life**.

The fragmentation of work or business interests includes no fixed form of work or study, temporary contracts (Justice) or **uncontracted work roles**.

However, the Fool-ish dissolution of barriers that prevent **the absorption of another personality can greatly benefit dramatic actors and performers** (Sun, KW, QW) or those acting out a role to feel more socially and culturally accepted (Hierophant) in the workplace. As an **underdeveloped, impressionistic, absorptive or half-formed personality**, the Fool's performances as others pro-vide them with an opportunity to feel whole and complete again (World), and thus can be highly convincing.

In addition, **the Fool-ishly playful and creative ego, which delights in dissolving order, shape and form, can produce great** abstract, impressionist or metaphysical artists and creatives (World, Empress, Magician, High Priestess). Their innocent, fantastical and otherworldly views (High Priestess, Magician, World, Empress) can capture the public imagination (Sun, Moon) by providing a pure impression of what lies beyond the material plane of existence.

Property – Finances – Resources

Carrying little material baggage or travelling light, the Fool often lives a minimalist lifestyle with few materialistic concerns, financial obligations or dependencies. Though they may not be materially wealthy, however, they can certainly qualify for the spiritually rich list.

As the archetype of beginnings, freedom and severance, the Fool can represent starting from scratch (1S, PP) and being materially and financially at (or back at) square one. They often don't know or care where their next pay cheque is coming from (PP), and unless they are independently wealthy (KP, QP, 10P), this lack of forethought will result in an erratic life, full of financial ups and downs (2P).

The Fool card may also indicate the receiving of severance pay (Death, 1S, 5P). Sometimes it can indicate relinquishing or leaving behind all material possessions (Hermit) and continually moving on from one place to the next, having given up a fixed address (KnW).

Knowing they are at the beginning of their journey, with not much to lose, can prompt this all-in archetype to take a big uncalculated risk with a speculative project or investment (Strength). Whether it pays off or not depends on the surrounding or outcome cards.

Health and Well-being

At their best, the Fool represents **youth or youthful energy and the vigour that comes from having an emotionally or physically lightened load. Hence this card is great if you are wanting to lose weight.**

Due to the archetype's **wide-open boundaries, the Fool is an adept at mediation practices (Temperance) and can easily find great solace, freedom and liberation from painful or stressful health concerns.**

However, **their carefree, complacent attitude to health and well-being is often only sustainable in the earlier years of life,** and can bring much trouble later on unless it is kept in check by the more health-conscious archetypes (Sun, Temperance, Star, High Priestess, Hierophant, Justice).

1 THE MAGICIAN I

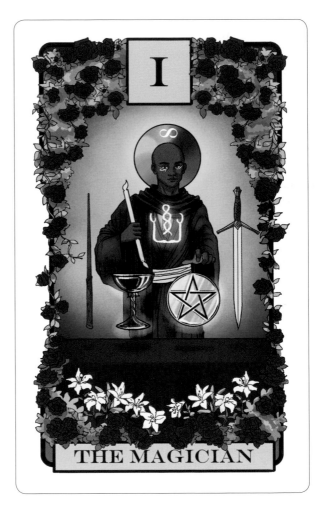

THE MAGICIAN

'It is a fine game to play, the game of politics,
and it is well worth waiting for a good
hand before really plunging.'
SIR WINSTON CHURCHILL

Personification – Psychology

The Magician is the master initiator of all opportunity and possibility (Aces). Their mode of consciousness, being ultra-agile, flexible, fertile and growth-oriented, i.e. growing away from the darkness (unless this is a layout crossing card) and towards the 'light', allows their experience of life to be positively infinite or unlimited.

The etymological line of 'magic', which stems from **magus, magi, imagery, imagination (Moon)**, reveals that **the source of the Magician's power is wholly mentalized.** Their **extraordinary mental skill (3P)**, particularly in **mastering such internally opposing forces as a rampant and intensive ego desire (Devil)**, is what ensures their success in all endeavours.

Empowered by their deep intrinsic understanding of how the world's systems work, the Magician skilfully implements this knowledge with the greatest possible, even magical, effect. Their judgement is even **resistant to modern 'scientifically' objective conditioning.** They don't allow themselves to be defined, as does the modern psyche, by 'me, myself, I' as opposed to 'it, that, you'. Where the modern psyche likes to 'know' where it begins and ends, **the magical psyche understands that 'beginning' and 'ending' are a material illusion; that, regardless of our distinctly different material hosts or vehicles, every living organism shares the same animating life-force energy.**

The fully enabled magical mode of consciousness is born of a deep and pervading connection to the surrounding world. **Seeing everything as an extension of itself, or more precisely as an energetic metaphor of its thoughts, it assumes personal ownership and ultimate responsibility for all its life events and encounters.**

When C. G. Jung shunned the modern cult of sense-perceptible science in his statement, '**I shall not commit the fashionable** stupidity [Fool, Pages] of regarding everything I cannot explain as a fraud,' he gave us a sense of how and why the magical mentality tends to be misunderstood and misrepresented. Unfortunately, **the all-pervasive subjectivity** of this archetype is all too often falsely likened to the blinkered experience of a psychological projection, purely because rational and logical thinkers cannot ground it in their concept of 'reality'. Yet the multi-dimensional magical mentality cannot be bound or limited by the confining presuppositions of third-dimensional 'realism'.

Spirituality and Philosophy

The Magician's clock-like hands, in their **'as above so below' position, point, literally and figuratively, to the heavenly eleventh hour, the hour of spiritual enlightenment,** and the opposite fifth hour, of material Earth challenges. The gesture suggests a divinely timed 'clockwork' connection between these two polar positions: **that great heavenly gifts come as a result of great earthly challenges, in an infinitely cyclical clock-like motion, pertaining to the cerebral cycles of spiritual development and even reincarnation.**

The Magician **controls the primitive, enlivening and vital life-force energy that gives birth to all sentient life,** whereas the Emperor, who comes second in the tarot's manifestation hierarchy, manages, directs and channels this energy into finite material and physical ambitions.

Having already learned and mastered their earthly lessons and transcended the drives, ambitions and desires of the ego (Emperor), the Magician works with an **all-pervading eleventh-hour state of consciousness to carry out the seemingly impossible in terms of the material and physical world.** By reconciling their base and selfish desires (Devil) with this **purer,**

brighter, innocent and selflessly enlightened consciousness, they become a truly clear energy channel and can overcome any material and physical limitations or restrictions. The full clarity of their words, deeds and actions enables a powerful alchemical transformation to take place, leading to full self-realization (High Priestess), spiritual maturation (Hermit), ego transcendence (Temperance) and self-healing (Star). This highly refined, spiritual state of consciousness is the primary prerequisite for the magical skill and ability to physically work 'reality' to their advantage (3P).

This archetype also has the singular ability to **bring forth shocking and powerful self-transformation.** Any conjoining 'agent' cards lend fuel to their **continually self-instigated process of growth, change and transformation,** and by relinquishing the past fully and completely, as if it never happened, they are able to embrace their newly empowered identity wholly and completely (World).

In their full harnessing of the immeasurable potential of a completely freed will, the Magician **personifies the most magical of our modern-day privilege empowerments.** The intensified concentration of sunlight through a magnifying glass illustrates how **their mastered mind accomplishes great things via its expansive, laser-like focus.**

The Magician's position as card number one is explained by the etymology of the word 'sorcery', which, coming from the Latin *sor, sorstis* or *sortiarius*, means **'one who influences lot, fate and fortune (by returning to the spiritual source of life itself)'.** In returning to the source, the Magician's **multidimensional mentality transcends the modern obsession with three-dimensional, sense-perceptible material fact.** As an adept of **supernatural skills and faculties (High Priestess, 3P),** the Magician can enact any passionately desired outcome via their **strong psycho-spiritual awareness.**

When this card appears in a reading, it is a time to **be ultra-careful what you wish for and guard against ungrounded wishful thinking (7C)**. Projecting negative, harmful or destructive ego intentions onto others in an attempt to control them (Devil) constitutes a truly self-defeating (5S) and self-destructive (10S) enactment of the Magician's power and influence. Psychically sending negative, harmful or destructive thoughts another person's way (Devil), even without acting on them, serves only to destabilize your own psycho-emotional health and happiness (Moon), which, paradoxically, then hands your power over to the very person you are seeking to disempower. Impure or negatively motivated desires (Devil) often come with a heavy hidden price attached.

When amongst friendly and constructive cards in a reading, this archetype indicates **your actions, words and deeds are wholly aligned, and so magically supported by the higher will of the Divine, the great universal architect, God or the forces of creation (whatever you wish to name it)**.

Personal Life

The Magician card represents **the 'heaven on earth' relationship (2C, 10C)**: that great heavenly gifts (1C, 2C, 10C) result from rising above the challenges of earthly life (Hermit, Tower, Death). It indicates **a magically transformative, alchemical union (2C, 10C) that is enlightening (Sun), a highly spiritual romance in which both parties are independently loving and detached from the ego.**

This card marks the **divinely magical and synchronized timing** by which two individuals come together, encounter each other for the first time (1C), and become romantically committed and entwined (2C). However, this archetype, being **primarily con-**

cerned with the sacred rather than mundane events of life, can be an inconsistent partner, providing great love-powered highs (Sun, 1C) and great insecurity-powered lows (Moon, Devil, Tower, 5P, 5C, 3S, 9S).

A relationship with the Magician archetype can be **enchanting, mesmerizing, fascinating, seductive (Lovers, Devil)** and **highly sexed (Emperor, 1W)**. They are often **a partner whose words have great power and influence over you (KS, QS)**. Under the influence of a negatively toned Magician (Devil), you can encounter a **highly manipulative or narcissistic individual**, bent on controlling others. The Magician can also be the ultimate **sexual predator (Devil)** who casts their 'wand' out (1W) and about in search of quick, self-serving gratification. If this card appears, it may be time for **a reality check to ensure others aren't taking advantage** of you.

Professional Life

The modern-day Magician's work life often deals with **matters pertaining to life, death or major transformation**. They appear at precisely the right time, as if your life and theirs are magically synchronized, and come in the form of **brilliant doctors, surgeons, life coaches, psychotherapists and psychiatrists, or even the executors of a last will and testament that leaves you a life-changing legacy (10P)**. They are the **pivotal movers, shakers and agents** who help secure your dream professional role.

By **holding all the aces**, the Magician represents **all new work and career avenues, advances and advantages**. When they are present in a work reading, you are likely to be in a **highly advantageous position (7W) or in line for a promotion (Emperor, Empress)**. Using their particular skills and abilities, the Magician also **excels in tests, examinations or interviews (Chariot)**. They often have a **powerful voice**, which they utilize in the manifesta-tion of their desires. They can be **a master spin doctor (Devil)** who harnesses the power of the spoken word to their own recondite ends, and they can utilize a vast amount of **hidden or camouflaged information (High Priestess)**, particularly regard-ing the timing of birth, death or transformation cycles within the work environment. They are **a formidable competitor (5W) who holds the professional life or death of others in their hands.**

The Magician's **complete self-mastery** is what ensures their great success in the external world at large, and due to their masterful reputation, they are also **someone people look to for magical solutions (8W)**. When working for the greater good, they can be key to **the miraculous unification (3C, Temperance)** of diametrically different groups of people or warring factions of a business sector or company (5W).

Property – Finances – Resources

'It's unlimited what the universe can bring when you
understand the great secret that thoughts become things.'
ANONYMOUS

Your positive expectations will be happily met, if not exceeded, when the Magician card appears in a finances reading, as, via the power of their mind, they **masterfully manifest** anything you might require in life. In a home this could be a water feature, pond, river, lake, beach, swimming pool (1C, KC, QC); a tradi-tional, period or 'des res' type property or location (1P, KP, QP); action and excitement in the heart of the city or a sporting, activity-based location (1W, KW, QW); and/or an intelligent or cutting-edge property design and mentally stimulating location (1S, KS, QS).

The Magician also represents **the settling of any material debts (Temperance)** or **the liquidating of any jointly held capital or assets in your favour (Justice)**. They have **a magical resourcefulness, a finger in every pie (World)**. **Their acquisitions and investments have infinite possibility and potential (World)**.

This is the archetype who **manifests great wealth and abundance (10P, KP, QP)**, **giving you everything you could ever need in life (Emperor, Empress)**.

Health and Well-being

The Magician represents the **attaining of great heavenly gifts (1C, High Priestess) as a result of great physical challenges, pain and suffering (Hermit)**. How long you must endure such challenges and difficulties depends; **working on philosopher René Descartes' principle 'I think therefore I am' (Moon)**, when the Magician's magically creative mind considers itself healthy and happy, it will be – instantaneously.

The Magician has **an uncanny ability to heal themselves both physically and emotionally using their infinite energetic reserves (KW, QW, KnW)** and **strong-willed initiative (Emperor)**. Their **authentic knowledge (High Priestess)** of how to maintain their health significantly lessens the chance of their contracting an illness or suffering a period of ill-health.

They are the archetype of **ultimate self-liberation** from unhealthy habits such as overeating or drinking. They have **controlled or balanced energies and hormones (Temperance)**, **with a strong and highly functioning immune system (Strength)**.

They also have **the power to create new life (1W, 1P, 1C)** and so represent male (Emperor) and female (Empress) fecundity, fertility and pregnancy, either naturally or via successful fertility treatments (8P).

2 THE HIGH PRIESTESS II

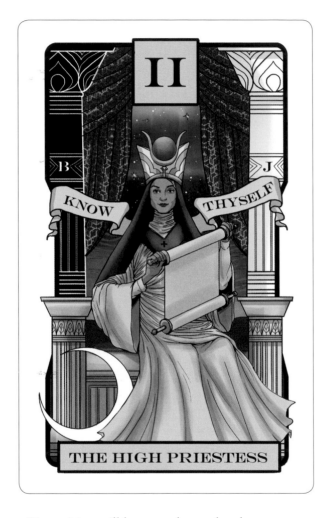

'Your vision will become clear only when you can
look into your own heart. Who looks outside,
dreams; who looks inside, awakes.'

C. G. JUNG

Personification – Psychology

In a similar way to the paradoxical and contradictory Moon, which is both inconstant and habitual, the High Priestess is an archetype concerned with both closure and disclosure, covering and discovering the ultimate or highest truth. They can provide piercing and incisive revelations (1S), while also being a trusted and faithful keeper of secret or hidden information. Good counsel or the true facts of a matter, legal (Justice) or otherwise, can come forth from hidden or not so obvious Priestess-type sources when this card appears. These sources are society's small or discreet 'aperture windows', both revealing and concealing the raw facts of hidden or subtle matters.

The High Priestess often has an exceptional sensitivity to hidden or subtle motivations (Devil, 7S), followed by a reflex tendency for counter-corrective words and actions (KnS), fired by a divinely inspired social transparency agenda (KS, QS).

The archetype is sincere and gracious, high-minded and intuitive in their reasoning, with great compassion for those stuck in a painful cerebral cycle and suffering from their base impulses and instincts. They see and understand what is incomprehensible in material world terms.

The High Priestess can be an inconspicuous force of good, operating behind the scenes (7S) and exerting great power and influence without being domineering. They can exert a subtle or hidden power over a person or situation, akin to how the Moon moves the tides, to bring about great and positive growth, change and transformation. As such, this card reveals by what hidden or obscured forces you are moved to action.

Privately and authentically, without seeking external ego recognition, praise or reward, the High Priestess also helps others reconcile and reintegrate any debased, degenerate, wild, animalistic ego tendencies (Devil) so they can live fuller and happier lives (Sun, 10C).

Spirituality and Philosophy

As a pure, exalted, gracious, maturely seeking and awakened consciousness, the High Priestess cuts through any superficial layers of experience and conditioning (1S) to reveal the **true self**, and thus is a key archetypal figure in the process of **major spiritual transformation (Magician).**

This archetype starts the psychical evaluation process that is so necessary for spiritual growth or progress via a general **illuminating, cleaning and clearing of the dark recesses and corners of the mind (Sun, Moon).** Through the Priestess's compassionate intervention, an individual can become **better acquainted with the unknown aspects of the self that keep them locked into ignorance and suffering.** 'Know Thyself', a phrase positioned high above the main entrance to the ancient Greek Temple of Apollo, **was the most highly regarded instruction of the infamous Delphic Oracles.** Still pertinent, it invites you to **explore your own mind as you would a temple.**

The High Priestess has a **dualistic, non-judgemental, all-encompassing mentality, rising above the world of opposites and polarities** – up and down, true and false, good and bad – and is **primarily inspired and instructed by ancient and obscured spiritual wisdom traditions (6C, Moon), and often party to the masonic-style secrets (3P) prohibited by conventional religions.** Similar to the Fool, the dissolution of the High Priestess's 'I think' and 'I know' ego operations echoes the Socratic paradox 'The only thing I know is that I know nothing.'

Portrayed in a womanly form, symbolizing the passive female principle, the High Priestess understands that **using the mascu-**

line ego-fired intellect alone without any input from the liquid-intuitive heart (3S) ultimately limits what you can achieve in life (8S).

By paying attention to anomalous information as it enters the mind, no matter how irrational, illogical and nonsensical, Priestesses **know exactly what, when, how and why, as their intuitive mind leaps over any slower cognitive processes.**

The key to the success of the High Priestess is in their overriding of the ego, which perceives **their inexplicable intuitions, instincts and gut feelings** as a threat to its position in the psychical hierarchy.

Characterized by their **far-reaching vision or foresight (3W, Star, World)**, the High Priestess has a **penetrative and omniscient mind. Whether divining the future or understanding the hidden truth of a current scenario,** they utilize a wide range of specialist skills and tools to **gain greater understanding of the subtle forces at work** in any given situation. These skills include **claircognizance, clairvoyance, clairaudience and clairsentience; the divination arts: tarot, astrology, psychic work, mediumship; out-of-body experiences, lucid dreaming; and dream, symbol and image interpretation (Empress, KS, QS).**

However, under the influence of impure (Devil), imaginary (Moon, 7C), immature, exaggerating (Pages), scattered or ungrounded (Fool) influences, this archetype can indicate being deceived by **false, inaccurate or self-fulfilling prophecies.**

Personal Life

In a relationship reading, the High Priestess represents a **deep, sincerity of feeling (KC, QC) devoid of any co-dependent or self-validating ego attachment (2C).** When this card appears, **showing your true complete self and sharing your innermost** thoughts and feelings with a trusted partner (2C) are paramount. This archetype is often deeply attuned to a partner's needs (2C) and their unions can feel sacred or tantric, spiritually connected or divinely inspired (1C).

The High Priestess can also indicate hidden or secret relationships (7S), where one or both parties are kept in the dark mentally, emotionally or even physically if there is a proverbial 'hidden woman' on the scene.

As is their dualistic nature, the High Priestess can represent either the hiding or revealing of 'closeted' romantic feelings, intentions or sexuality. Being ruled by the Moon, they can symbolize cyclical romantic feelings that 'come and go', ebb and flow, as the Moon moves the tides (Lovers, Moon).

If you are single and seeking a partner, this archetype can sometimes indicate the meeting of a new love interest (1C, KnC) via spiritual friends and connections (3C).

Professional Life

The High Priestess represents those whose work life is devoted to compassionately bettering the lives of others, helping them realize and actualize their fullest possible potential (World). They often work from home or behind the scenes, working nights (Moon) or undercover, perhaps as super-sleuths, detectives (Justice), in espionage, with hidden surveillance systems (Star), in the intelligence services (KS, QS), in hidden, secretive or sensitive work, or investment speculations (Strength), as futurologists predicting economic or market trends (World), as researchers (KC, QC) or archivists (6C, Moon), in counter-cultural, fringe or taboo-themed industries, as spiritual teachers and mentors (Hierophant), counsellors, life coaches, psychotherapists, spiritual advisers (KC, QC) or well-being or spiritual events facilitators (3C, Hierophant).

This archetype, which delights in highlighting cultural corners and edges, can even work for counter-cultural, grassroots, fringe organizations, or any sector beyond the tight, spotlit sphere of centralized comprehension and experience (Sun).

Wherever it happens to be, whereas the Magician is the active, masculine power behind the throne, the High Priestess works predominantly in hidden or passive power positions. They are the office or employer's confidante, the person who knows, but never shares, what is going on behind the scenes (7S). Due to their secret partnerships or alliances (2W, 2C) they are often in and out of covert or secretive talks and meetings (3W, 3C).

This 'left of field' archetype stays on top (7W) by obtaining their information or ideas via rare, unusual, eccentric, out of the box, unconventional or inaccessible sources or methods. They possess rare skills, talents or knowledge that can either be feared (9S) or celebrated (Sun) and sought after by others (3P). Yet their subtle work efforts can be easily eclipsed or overlooked when they are competing with more mainstream or commanding personalities (Emperor, Empress, KW, QW). However, the sometimes torpid world of work can be shaken out of its stupor (4S, 4C) by the Priestess's exotic, fascinating, unusual, unconventional and non-conformist approach.

Flanked by high-visibility influences (Sun, World), the truth, wisdom and insight of this archetype, portrayed in obscure, unconventional, private, fantastical, otherworldly (World, 7C), underworld or taboo themes, is likely to celebrated and well received (Sun, 3P).

Property – Finances – Resources

Being spiritually inclined, the High Priestess can signify **unmaterialistic living** with few financial obligations, commitments or dependants and an impartial attitude to money and resources (Fool).

They may or may not be materially rich, depending on the surrounding cards, but instead have **immaterial or spiritual wealth and riches in abundance (1C, 10C)**. Akin to the wandering ascetics, nuns or monks, the Priestess **often attains unlimited access (Fool) to their spiritual gifts in those times when material resources are voluntarily renounced (Hermit) or involuntarily limited (5P)**.

Unless influenced by more social (3C, 3W, 3P) or high-visibility (Sun, World) cards, the High Priestess indicates **buying land or property in a quiet or largely unfrequented place**.

When flanked by other benevolent cards, they tend to **put earned material abundance towards altruistic acts of charity (World, 6P)**, doing what they perceive as the right thing (Justice) regardless of personal cost.

When flanked by a malefic (Devil) or miserly (4P) card, they can represent **the concealing or sudden discovery of secretly hidden wealth and resources**.

Health and Well-being

As the earthly vehicle of the soul, the High Priestess **worships and respects their body and mind as they would a religious house or sacred temple (Sun)**. However, **a person under the influence of this archetype can also lose sight of the true earthly purpose of life, their sacred outlook rendering them blind to the** necessary counter-balancing effects of an ordinary life (Moon, 4C).

When influenced by benevolent cards, the High Priestess can serve themselves and others by **using their insight and divinatory skills for the purposes of self- or soul-realization: unburdening or 'en-lightening' the mind and spirit of mundane concerns (Sun).**

Influenced by cards pressing a shadow agenda (Devil), however, the High Priestess can be prone to **hidden or secret obsessions and addictions.** Their **passive attitude to exercise,** which ebbs and flows like the tides, can be the cause of any health or well-being issues.

Sometimes this card can indicate **a hidden or undiagnosed health issue,** but more often it indicates **a deep, intuitive understanding of any health or well-being imbalances.**

Regardless of whether they are active (Wands, Swords) or inactive (Pentacles, Cups), **this night-owl archetype may suffer from a vitamin D deficiency or other imbalances connected to a lack of exposure to sunlight.**

Being the archetype of openings, this card can also represent **health issues involving the nine aperture windows of the body.** It can also indicate **the decision to conceal the news of an illness or pregnancy (Empress, 1C, 1W),** perhaps only until the end of the first trimester.

3 THE EMPRESS III

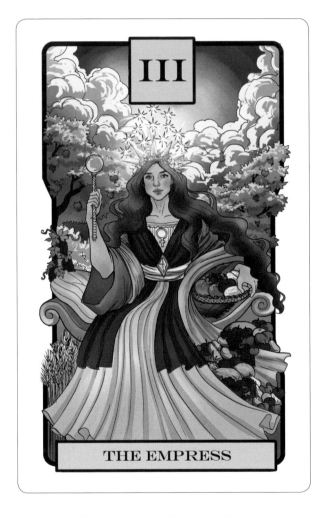

THE EMPRESS

'Allow yourself to be beautiful and
all the rest will follow.'
THE BUDDHA

Personification – Psychology

The Empress is **a vivacious character who personifies charm, grace, beauty, creativity or fertility (Sun)**. Empresses are dedicated to nurturing and nourishing others and making them feel good about themselves, and so are often greatly valued, loved and respected.

Their social identity can be either **the well-regarded or highly creative woman or the primary matriarchal guardian, mother or mother figure, whose self-validation (Sun) or sense of wholeness and completion (World) derives solely from their physical fertility and reproductive accomplishments (Pages)**.

Mother figure or not, Empresses experience **great life satisfaction and often share their good fortune with others, whom they treat with great kindness, love and affection, which is key to the Empress's inner and outer success.**

The Empress's primary concerns in life are **love, happiness and harmony; marriage, love-making, enjoyment, amusement, charm, delights, pleasures, pleasantries, deliciousness, sugary or indulgent food, fine wines, art, design, creativity, music, concerts, dance, dancing parties, sociability, sensual pleasure, perfume, scents, decorations and ornaments, all forms of comfort and prosperity promotion, accumulated wealth, ornamentation, fine clothes and accessories, jewels, gems, precious stones, make-up, beauty, fashion and womanly products and experiences.**

The Empress's complete immersion in **the joys of life and unrelenting pursuit of pleasure and sensual fulfilment (9C, 10C)** are often experienced in **highly civilized or agreeable surroundings (9P, 10P)**. Unless flanked by destructive cards (Tower, Death, 3S), the Empress is **a maker of relationships – one who listens, appreciates, unconditionally accepts, understands and responds to others' needs (6P)**.

While some archetypes devote their time and energy to the forceful **pursuit of rule and domination (Emperor)**, the Empress **rules and dominates via attraction (Lovers) and accommodation (Temperance).** Chinese strategist and philosopher of the Zhou dynasty Sun Tzu once wrote, '**Success is gained by carefully accommodating ourselves to the enemy's purpose,**' which gives an idea of how we might effectively apply Empress energy to contentious, difficult or challenging situations. Indeed, the highest, purest expression of this energy, in which the archetype wields the greatest power and influence, can be seen in all the Empress's **loving, kind and tender-hearted words and actions, motives and agendas.**

However, **if the Empress is all heart and no head, they can overindulge or be too obliging to those around them. Also, sometimes the Empress themselves can be spoilt by having had too much of a good thing, and so be prone to a kind of 'gilded cage' syndrome, where lethargy, boredom, laziness and procrastination (4C) rule their thinking.**

Undoing any fixed expectation or deeper sense of entitlement (Moon, 1S) often involves much pain and suffering, so the higher the ego climbs (Sun, KW, QW), the harder it falls for this elevated archetype (Tower). If left unchecked, the Empress's **pretentions, pride, prejudice, vanity or queenly behaviour can be their downfall (Tower, Death, 10S).** Marie Antoinette, the last queen of France, made such a *faux pas*, which cost her her life, when she replied to a call from her starving people for more bread with '**Let them eat brioche.**' Whether these were her actual words or political anti-monarchic spin, **the queen's past vanity, prejudice and pretentions gave the people cause to believe her capable of saying them.**

Spirituality and Philosophy

Being primarily concerned with the superficial, material or sensual aspects of life (KP, QP, KnP), **the Empress can have only skin-deep spiritual awareness.** However, this archetype's **core spirituality can be excavated and expressed via creative pursuits and endeavours.**

By remaining **out of touch with harsh, unpleasant or obscured realities, such as the poverty of others,** the Empress puts themselves at a spiritual disadvantage, though, for their rose-tinted outlook **makes it difficult for this archetype to look at or confront their own unlikeable shadow aspects.**

Unless more active and assertive cards are present (Emperor, KW, QW, 10W, KS, QS), this **wholly passive archetype always takes the path of least resistance in life.** However, in their internal battle to subdue and integrate the ego, their passive approach does have a key spiritual role to play. 'The supreme art of war is to subdue the enemy without fighting' is Sun Tzu's description of the Empress's **application of the passive female principle to bypass male ego-activated intentions.**

Thus the Empress's influence can help us accomplish great spiritual feats when we allow things to happen by simply **tuning into the vital life-force energies that surround us, rather than attempting to own and control them with our ego.**

Personal Life

The Empress indicates **mature, sincere, unconditional love and acceptance, romance and attraction; a diplomatically balanced and harmoniously allied marriage or relationship (2C, 10C); feeling loved, irresistible, worshipped and adored; having several** admirers (8W) or sensual fun and pleasure providers (KnP, KnC, 2P); overflowing with sweet and sincere feelings (1C); providing emotional comfort and security (10C); sweet, deep, true love and commitment in relationships (2C, 10C); someone looking out for you, making sure all your wants, needs and desires are fulfilled; a very pleasant, loving, caring, content or rewarding relationship (9C).

As a partner, the Empress can be highly appealing, attractive, sexual, fertile, delightful, charming, elegant, virtuous, graceful, polished, refined, cultured and liberally minded, with strong, exalted feminine graces or highly civilized feminine values.

The Empress is the agent of **magnetic attractiveness, charm, passive possessiveness and incoming energy,** used both consciously and unconsciously to draw in a mate (2C) or to matchmake for others (Magician). In its most positive expression, this archetype signifies the wife, the committed mate (2C) and those in counselling and advising roles, such as friends, family or professional marriage or relationship counsellors (High Priestess, KC, QC) who help to strengthen partnerships.

In its most challenging expression, the Empress represents smothering or motherly lovers (Lovers, Moon) or the limitations and restrictions (8S) of searching for **a true heart connection** (1C, 2C) when moving only in the small social circles of the highly privileged few. When partners fail to meet the Empress's status, class or wealth standards, this archetype needs to assess whether allowing their **emotional comfort to be affected by social or material concerns** really is the true path to love and happiness.

As a layout crossing card, this archetype can indicate, for both men and women, the selecting of an ultra-attractive life partner, either due to their looks, wealth or status, as a form of **self-flattery**. Unless a couple's love can grow, change and penetrate further than merely skin deep, over time, when this attractive and flattering mirror image of the self begins to show its illusionistic and transitory nature, the 'love spell' will fracture and eventually break (Lovers, Tower).

Professional Life

Whether meeting the **highest outward standards or keeping up appearances**, the Empress indicates great success in the broadly creative industries: home comforts, family planning (3P), parenting, business deals, negotiation, diplomacy, creativity, art and design, literature, entertainment, high-end leisure or luxury services, beauty, femininity, nature, farming and fruitfulness in food, flora, fauna production (7P).

This archetype can indicate **a flourishing business or much-admired project**, even the best in show or a showpiece. Being the centre of attention, on display for all to see and admire (Sun), the Empress can also represent fashions, trends, image-conscious professions, branding and advertising (8W).

By their highly creative endeavours and infectious passion for their work (KW, QW), the Empress reaches the top of their game and can be rewarded with a vastly upgraded office space or work environment (4W), a highly desired new position (Aces) or the exceptional success of their product (World). Their creative efforts tend to have universal or mass appeal (Sun). They can be super-successful in **all aesthetics-based businesses or industries** where an appreciation of good looks, charm, an amiable personality, dressing to impress, beauty or style are the keys to getting ahead or commanding the attention of others (Sun, KW, QW). As such, this archetype can also represent **ego and vanity projects** (Devil, Sun), which exist superficially or only for show (Sun).

When flanked by positive, friendly and harmonious cards, the Empress's work can bring great joy and contentment **to the lives of others**. Though it doesn't constitute a basic survival need, **their sphere of work can make people's lives feel all the richer, as argued by the painter Pablo Picasso when he said, 'You know, music, art – these are not just little decorations to make life prettier. They're very deep necessities which people cannot live without.'**

Property – Finances – Resources

The Empress can be **an excellent provider, both of finances and resources (10P), and this card's presence in a reading signifies great material success: the proverbial harvest coming in.** Being a feminine archetype, this is the card of **passive earning: it symbolizes a harvest time, when you reap the rewards of your previous hard work or past efforts.**

The Empress can also be **charitable and generous** in sharing personal wealth and resources (6P), but must remain astute lest their **passive and obliging nature** is taken advantage of by others (Devil).

This archetype can represent living **the 'charmed' life of a kept or independently wealthy individual, living off unearned family money, a trust fund or their partner's income (KP, QP, 10P).** If this is the case, look to the surrounding cards to see if this is a blessing or a hindrance to their overall personal happiness and sense of fulfilment. Chronic boredom (4C) can result from being handed everything with little or no effort. Also, if cards of delusion are present, this archetype's **sense of privilege or entitlement** can be wholly imagined (Moon, 7C) and unfounded (Fool).

Health and Well-being

Being comfort oriented, the Empress can be **prone to laziness or excessive passivity (4S)**; however, this card is a blessing for those who find it difficult to relax, rest and unwind, and is of particular benefit during trying or stressful times. It often signifies **some form of retreat or well-deserved time off (4S)**, a time of feeling wholly **nourished (Star)** after a great effort or exertion.

During the passive Empress period, your **emotional (Cups), mental (Swords), physical (Wands) and material (Pentacles)** balance and harmony can be fully replenished and restored **(Temperance)**. This is therefore the ideal time for **natural conception or success with fertility treatments, which will be likely to result in a pregnancy (1C, 1W, 1P) and childbirth (Pages)**.

4 THE EMPEROR IV

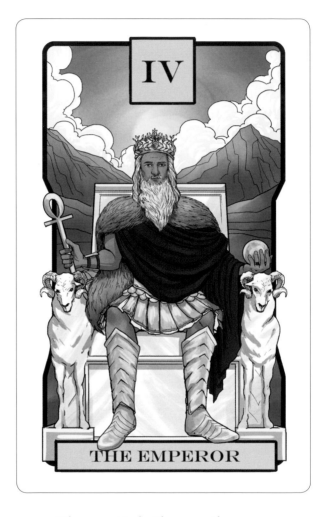

'The expert in battle moves the enemy,
and is not moved by him.'
SUN TZU

Personification – Psychology

The Emperor archetype **likes to be first and foremost or** given primacy and priority to retain their leading position (7W). Their primary drive or impulse to **arrive first or lead the way extends to initiating, founding, pioneering, newness, novelty, innovation, invention, individuality, originality and uniqueness (Aces).** The US Supreme Court Justice (Emperor, Justice) Antonin Scalia, aka **the 'Originalist',** once retold the story of two guys who were out hunting when a bear started chasing them. They started running, but the bear was gaining fast. One said, 'Why are we running? We can't outrun a bear.' And the other said, 'I don't have to outrun the bear, I only have to outrun you.' This is **the survivalist mindset** of the tarot's Emperor archetype.

The Emperor's quest is to **find and propound great new theories or potential (Star, Aces), seek new horizons (KnW) and be at the forefront, driving, moving or leading the flock, herd, team, group or troop.**

As the archetype of our primary life-force vitality, the Emperor manages, channels, aims and directs it into either material resources (Pentacles), love and feelings (Cups), physical acts (Wands) or intellectual interests (Swords).

In opposition to their Empress counterpart, the Emperor **thrives on challenge, and will often take the path of most resistance** (10W). They aim for **the mark of excellence and the highest possible professional achievement in their personal or work endeavours (World, Sun).** As such, **their sense of self-worth and ego validation is often solely reliant on their outward successes and achievements.** This can, unless consciously processed, set them up for huge blows (Tower) to their self-esteem and confidence (8S, 9S, 10S) when they experience any sort of failure, be it material (Pentacles), emotional (Cups), mental (Swords) or physical (Wands).

A destabilized, negatively toned Emperor who has perhaps received a blow to their pride or self-esteem can display **exaggerated masculinity, will-power, selfishness, chauvinism, supremacy and defensive invulnerability (9W, KNW, KNS)** or behaviour that is **overpowering, domineering, high-handed, oppressive, opinionated, dictating, forceful, controlling, bossy, strict, authoritarian and even persecuting, intimidating, stubborn, unyielding, obstinate and inflexible.** Yet in the appropriate context, this archetype's rigidity can be key to their success.

Under stabilizing influences (Hermit, Hierophant, Empress, Judgement), the Emperor can display **solid reasoning and judgement, extraordinary self-control, patience and persistence, a reasonable nature, and astute, intelligent and worldly thinking and decision-making (World, KS, QS, KnS).** Under higher-minded influences, they are capable of **great self-realization (High Priestess), conscious awareness (Sun), grounding (Hermit) and humility (Temperance).**

The Emperor has **great organizing ability and knows how to get the best out of others, be they family, friends or co-workers.** They have **strong parental and authoritarian instincts, born of an inherent capacity for home rule.** The cards surrounding this archetype in a reading will indicate whether their parenting style is working for them or not.

The ultimate example of the Emperor archetype is perhaps film director and father of seven Steven Spielberg, who once said, 'Fathering is a major job, but I need both things in my life – my job to be a director and my kids to direct me.' Spielberg's words are a great reminder that **behind the Emperor's throne there is often a strong directive, purpose or person(s) that empowers their otherwise self-directed actions.**

Spirituality and Philosophy

Unless a spiritual bent is indicated (Fool, Magician, High Priestess, Hierophant), the Emperor archetype can be **devoid of faith or belief in the subtle realms of the lesser known or seen**, especially as these challenge their cutting-edge or leading world view based upon the modern cult of scientific materiality and sense-perceptible 'fact' (KP, QP, KNP).

Unless neighbouring cards suggest a heightened conscious awareness or sensitivity to the subtle, spiritual and metaphysical realities (Sun, Moon, High Priestess, Magician, KC, QC), **that which appears illogical, irrational or materially inexplicable is anathema to the Emperor.** They aren't devoid of **subtle perception**, for they can read and appreciate fine art (KS, QS), for example, but the deeper spiritual forces (High Priestess) behind creative processes can elude them completely.

As the archetype who most appreciates masculine, tangible, material rewards and achievements (KP, QP), it often takes a great blow to the Emperor's ego, resulting in the greater self-realization that induces a spiritual awakening (Sun, Magician, High Priestess), for them to overcome their psycho-spiritual blocks and resistance.

Personal Life

A positively influenced Emperor denotes **honour, respect, protection, longevity, stability and monogamy in love, marriage and any other relationship** (2C, 4W, Hierophant).

As the epitome of **the protective male ego**, the psycho-emotional well-being of the Emperor archetype (Moon) relies on their not only being needed and useful as a partner, but also worshipped and adored (Sun, KW, QW). Emperors are often dutiful, dependable, responsible, influential and highly regarded by their partners; their final word, on almost all subjects, being generally accepted and followed. As such, the all-knowing, controlling, possessive, domineering, commanding, patriarchal or motive forcefulness of this archetype – telling you what to do and when to do it or setting out what they see as acceptable behaviour – is often behind any long-standing relationship politics (5W).

Paradoxically, it's the Emperor's ultra-masculine charm and optimism that first attracts the opposite sex (Lovers). They often make exceptionally virile lovers (1W), even when this card signifies an older partner or significant age gap.

Beyond their better, wiser judgement, this archetype holds rigidly to any perceived challenge or 'mountain' yet unclimbed. Their instigating, initiating, prize-winning, 'me-first' attitude to romance and relationships finds the initial pursuit, challenge or sexual conquest highly engaging (KnW, KnC, 9C), but then they can lose interest once the 'prize' is won (KnW).

For a harmonious love or marital life, this archetype tends to prefer an ultra-feminine and compliant Empress type whose own male energies are especially well regulated, allowing them to bend to the Emperor's will. For those who enjoy the traditional feminine role (Empress), the Emperor can be the perfect complementary partner. The modern, outgoing, high-achieving Superwoman type, being an Emperor in woman's clothing, is likely to encounter a 'battle of wills' with an Emperor-like partner, which leaves the latter feeling unfortunately emasculated.

Nonetheless, the Emperor's wilful and indomitable spirit can, under certain influences, be emotionally subdued, softened, coordinated and feminized (Moon, Temperance, KC, QC) to balance the stresses and strains of a high-performance masculine work life.

Professional Life

The Emperor is the primary archetype for **the attainment of a high, powerful or privileged position, public status, professional reputation and recognition.** They often thrive in competitive or combative environments (5W) where their formidable business skills take them to the very heights of an organization. They can be the managing force behind the chart topper, blockbuster or majorly successful project or product (10P, World), the ones at the top of the game, pulling the strings or initiating great new movements or revolutions (Aces, World).

This archetype reaches the top as CEO, commander, director, manager, conductor, captain, line manager or overseer due to sustained, consistent and persistent effort (8P): their practice made perfect. However, this can come at the expense of their mental and emotional health. The **workaholic** (10W) Emperor can suffer from extreme psychological stress (Moon) due to their restless preoccupation with business, action, achieving, attaining, doing, making, performing, exercise (10W, KW, QW) and strong aversion to idleness or inertia.

In their hot pursuit of perfection (8P), this archetype must guard against their behaviour becoming overly pushy, controlling, authoritarian or micromanaging (4P), lest they alienate their co-workers or convolute the proceedings.

Also, the Emperor, as a non-subordinate character with a strong aversion to being controlled, has a tendency to crush the opposition, which often puts them at the centre of any internal office or company politics (5W).

This is the archetype that **strives towards total self-sufficiency, self-employment, owning their own business or at the very least being employed at the very top of a command chain, so they always call the shots.**

The **highly respected** Emperor archetype usually has much expertise and experience in their particular field or arena (3P) and **an excellent reputation for getting results.** Their expertise extends to all forms of **dynamic business management, directing or producing.**

By always moving forward and embracing all that is foreign, exotic or unfamiliar, they are often the first to discover or open up uncharted sectors, markets and territories (Chariot). When something is about to have a moment (Sun, World), they are there, ready and prepared. They understand the movement of dynamic energies and thus make for an exceptional inventor and innovator in all fields where new ideas or new social movements break with outdated conventions (Judgement, Fool, Aces).

Being an archetypal outgoing 'because of' character, the Emperor can also press on (Chariot) and expand the scope of an operation beyond what anyone could have imagined or thought possible (World).

Property – Finances – Resources

As a **materially driven** archetype whose home is their 'castle' (KP, QP), the Emperor is **an ultra-reliable source of physical protection and financial security, with excellent future prospects** (KP, QP, 10P).

The Emperor card can even indicate **a generous patron, benefactor or provider** (6P), a solid long-term investment (10P) or the financial rewards from consistent work efforts (8P). If there have been any recent economic or financial setbacks (Death, Tower, 5P), the Emperor is more likely than any other archetype to initiate a quick and effective recovery.

The Emperor represents those in charge of any financial assets, such as land, property, stocks, bonds or an investment portfolio. They can be trusted to handle money matters carefully, with business-like restraint (Temperance).

However, as the archetype defined by what they can or can't accumulate, unless money matters are dealt with superconsciously (Sun, High Priestess), the Emperor's pursuit of ever-grander socio-material status can end up owning their life (KP, QP, 4P).

Health and Well-being

The Emperor's high vitality and managerial ability can lead them into captaining or leading a sports team, fitness or well-being group, though their drive to get ahead of others often leads to headaches, migraines or head-related injuries.

The Emperor represents all self-determined forms of growth, change and transformation (Magician, Wheel of Fortune), such as can result from dietary restrictions, limitations and intermittent fasting (Hermit). However, when flanked by unbalanced or disharmonious cards (5W), this archetype can symbolize not enough variety or fluids in the diet, resulting in a slow metabolism, digestion and constipation (Hanged Man, 4S, 8S).

Liking things their own way, this is the archetype most prone to ignoring the advice of social, health and well-being professionals (7W, 2S, 8S). The degree of their stubbornness, whether minor or acute, is often reflected in the stiffness, rigidity or inflexibility of their body and movement range (Hermit, 4P, 4S). Yoga or gymnastic exercise may help to finally free them, mind and body.

5 THE HIEROPHANT V

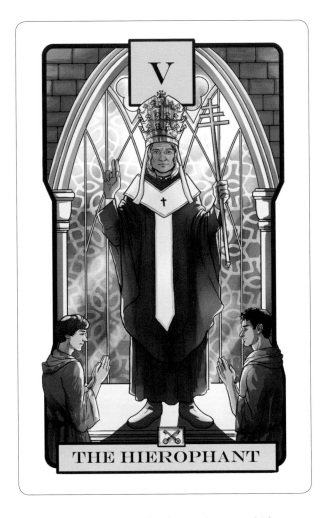

'The teacher who is indeed wise does not bid you to
enter the house of his wisdom but rather leads
you to the threshold of your mind.'

KHALIL GIBRAN

Personification – Psychology

This can be a joyous card for **those who relish an opportunity for deeper study (PP) or a scholastic life (KS, QS)**, but for the more outgoing (KW, QW) or free-spirited individual (Fool, Chariot, Sun), the Hierophantic life may feel boring (4C) or restrictive (Hanged Man, 8S).

This archetype is **primarily concerned with self-development, self-improvement and righting the wrongs of others.** They have **a mature and improving character, which is grateful, thankful, reverent, humble, penitent, remorseful, conscience-stricken and repentant.** Unless corrupted by cards indicating an ego objective or hidden agenda (Devil), the Hierophant's personal bent tends towards selflessness, altruism, humanity, clemency, benevolence, peace, harmony, doing the right thing and goodwill to all.

Doing unto others what they would have them do unto themselves, their approach to all situations is often well-meaning. As such, this archetype reflects an individual's relationship to social morality and charity, and their compassionate concern and willingness to guide and assist others (6P).

The Hierophant is characterized by their **restraint, discipline, self-control, higher integrity, sensible instruction, guidance and advice.** The card indicates a situation where **a formal, sincere, principled, conventional or traditional approach is taken towards life or business.**

Unless more progressive or unusual influences (Aces, Fool, Magician, High Priestess) appear, this **intransient** archetype tends to stick to what they know and is **reluctant to acknowledge or embrace any new or different cultural habits or belief systems (Moon).** However, by leading a **predictable, habitual, dogmatic, fixed and largely unvarying life (Moon),** the

Hierophant rarely destabilizes the status quo by any random or surprising behaviour.

Shaped, moulded or guided by longstanding traditions and regulatory institutions, the Hierophant religiously sticks to their path, honours their word and often gives their entire life over to a particular group or social cause. Yet, as a proponent of social or cultural norms, expectations, conventions, rules and regulations, they may find their knowledge and wisdom shunned by more headstrong, autonomous or self-regulating individuals (Emperor, Sun, KW, QW, KnW).

Whether instilled by community or family members, the Hierophant's **bureaucratic, ultra-traditional, conservative** or heavily conformist restrictions can feel like **a form of self-sacrifice or self-denial, where individual confidence is restricted or reduced (8S)**. The more radical and individualized (Fool, Magician, High Priestess, Sun) a person's mode or style of social self-expression (Sun), the more the Hierophant's **regulating code of conduct and social framework can feel like a strict schooling of thought (Moon)**. Thus Hierophant-style parenting (Emperor, Empress) can seem **old-fashioned or based on outdated principles**.

This is the archetype most likely to identify with **past cultural or religious traditions**, especially those that have spanned many centuries (Moon). It can also indicate the sense of belonging (Moon, 9C, 10C) to **a cultural group, society, club, association, spiritual or religious order, and forming a strong bond with a particular commercial brand, or a band of like-minded cultural brothers or sisters** (3C, 3W, 3P).

In some way or another, this archetype indicates a need for **structured authority and disciplined leadership: having either something or someone to follow. As an instructive archetype, the Hierophant often feels a need to lead others (Emperor, Sun), as well as being led themselves by a higher guiding principle, source or power.**

It is not unusual to find this archetype flanked by cards denoting emotionally desperate, vulnerable (5C, 5P), weak-minded, highly reflective, absorptive or easily influenced characters (Fool, Moon, Pages, 7C), who naturally seek out the guidance and teachings of stronger and more authoritative individuals. Unfortunately, unless it is flanked by more discerning and discriminatory cards (Magician, High Priestess, Emperor, Empress, Strength, Temperance, Kings/Queens), **the Hierophant's teachings can potentially be underdeveloped and misleading.**

The negatively toned (Devil), vulnerable, wounded or desperate Hierophant (Death, Tower, 3S, 5C, 5P, 5S, 5W), motivated by their own self-serving ego agenda (Emperor, Knights, Pages), **often attempts to convert naïve or weaker minds (Fool, Pages) to their way of thinking.** They are the influential friend, family member, romantic partner, indoctrinator, programmer, trainer, teacher or mentor who holds great sway or power over their child, lover, partner, student or follower, rendering them completely co-dependent, incapable of developing, maturing, thinking, acting or fending for themselves (8S, Pages).

Spirituality and Philosophy

The Hierophant can be a **spiritual way-shower (Magician, High Priestess)** who teaches, mentors or lectures on occluded, occult, hidden, underworld, secret and esoteric subjects. They can be **ambassadorial figures for the world's many and varied spiritual belief systems, whether associated with still-active faith religions or ancient power sources grounded in a knowledge of subtle extrasensory reality (Magician, High Priestess).**

This archetype represents a **true, complete, unwavering faith or devotion to a spiritual, religious or philosophical path. They** are ambassadors for what they believe in and remain strong in the face of any external objection or dissent (7W).

Unless supported by maturely questioning and discerning cards in a reading (Magician, High Priestess, Hermit, KS, QS), this archetype can represent those with a blind or blinkered devotion to a spiritual or religious leader (Moon, 2S, 8S) and those who allow themselves to be misled by the impure ego agenda of others (Fool, Devil).

Unless otherwise indicated by the presence of more free-thinking, original and creative cards (Fool, Magician, High Priestess, Empress), this archetype tends towards past imitations (Fool, Moon), copying what was done previously rather than adapting their approach to the modern mentality. As such, they tend to be primarily concerned with the continuation of historical practices and wisdom lineages via the study and teaching of ancient texts.

Personal Life

Due to the Hierophant's pack mentality, their close associations, be they friendships or partnerships, are often with like-minded individuals. As a partner, the Hierophant appeals to those looking for a conventional or traditional partnership that conforms exactly to society's expectations.

This archetype represents the continuance of ancient cultural traditions, such as marriage (Justice, 4W, 2C, 3C) or any other sacred vow, ceremony or ritual executed in a 'by the book' fashion, unless more creative (Empress) or radically self-expressive (Sun, Magician, KW, QW) influences are present.

At its most extreme spiritual expression, this archetype can represent sexual abstinence or celibacy (Strength, Hermit). This can be a by-product of the impulse to give up life's pleasures to follow a great spiritual (High Priestess, KC, QC) or scholarly passion (KS, QS).

Unless neighbouring cards suggest otherwise, this archetype's **rigidly structured or routine lifestyle habits can lack spontaneity, originality and creativity.** On a date, for example, they may opt for the safest choice, eating and drinking the same thing every time. Yet, like a spiritual passion or faith religion, **they can be someone who brings an inexplicable sense of meaning and purpose to their partner's life.**

When flanked by challenging or disruptive cards (5W, 5S, 5P, 5C), **the student–teacher dynamic of the partnership may have created a power imbalance.** Though revered by others for their learning and wisdom, worshipping or putting a Hierophantic partner on a pedestal (Sun), or even becoming overly fascinated (Devil) with them, can lead to a disempowering relationship dynamic.

However, when flanked by benevolent cards, this archetype represents the **sacred, reverent, balanced and unwavering love and loyalty (1C, 2C)** of a selflessly giving or helpful partner, **completely dedicated to their partner's happiness and well-being (10C, KC, QC).**

Professional Life

This archetype's positive sense of self-worth and self-validation (Sun) usually comes from **executing some form of social duty or making a significant contribution to community welfare.** The focus is on enriching the lives of their followers, clients, co-workers or employees, helping them to alleviate suffering and make peace with their lives.

The Hierophant is the highly regarded and inspiring **guru, mentor, teacher, professor, lecturer, instructor, orator, public** speaker or storyteller, the purveyor of wisdom teachings whose higher knowledge or philosophy (Sun) comes from scholarly (KS, QS), religious or spiritual sources (High Priestess).

When flanked by other major archetypes (Emperor, Empress, Magician, High Priestess) in a reading, it is likely that **you yourself are imparting some form of higher wisdom or knowledge to others. When the Hierophant is flanked by the court cards, you may feel inspired to attend another tutor, teacher or mentor's lecture (7W), class, course or workshop (8P).**

As a potential proponent of emotionally indoctrinating narratives, stories or allegories, the Hierophant's **cleverly instructive energy** (KS, QS) can be used to great effect in sales (2P), advertising and marketing (8W). Thus, when **the archetype of instruction** appears in a reading, extra diligence may be required to discern whether any impure motives or agendas (Devil) lie behind the information on offer.

This archetype can also represent **being initiated into the ranks of a company or organization that adheres to strict or highly disciplined, conventional or traditional ways of operating.** Unless influenced by flexible or changeable cards (Fool, Wheel of Fortune, 2P, Pages), **this archetype often sticks with the same, safe, secure and familiar type of work (Moon), and strictly conforms to their employers', colleagues', students' and own expectations.** The Hierophant can therefore be **an old or immovable source of power at the head of a longstanding organization, or, conversely, someone who historically had it all, but whose power and influence are not what they used to be (5C, 5S, 5P).**

Property – Finances – Resources

This archetype usually has their greatest success in **following time-tested or conventional methods of money-making and spending (KP, QP, KNP)**, and so rarely takes risks or does anything out of the ordinary with financial investments or property purchases.

This is the archetype of **conventional or even old-fashioned values**, particularly when it comes to who pays for a dinner date, or even who is the main provider or breadwinner (KP, QP, 10P).

Unless inflected by more wayward influences (Devil, 7S, 4P), this archetype usually **follows a strict moral compass** when it comes to making money and paying their dues. If someone has strayed from a straightforward or conventional course of action in their financial dealings, this card can represent a moral lesson, especially when dealing with legal, governmental or tax issues (Justice).

A hard lesson could have led to a reduced state of wealth and abundance (Hermit, 5P), which allows only those purchases that are absolutely necessary. The Hierophant can also represent voluntary austerity measures, religiously denying yourself any luxuries and indulgences.

This is the archetype of **providing time or money for charitable causes (6P)** or receiving monies and/or resources from those who believe or have faith in your longstanding project or cause. Like the modern-day Church, you may be **asset rich but cash poor (4P)**. A diminished or waning sense of financial power or control (Tower) may lead you to refocus your acquisition efforts away from the physical and material and towards spiritual wealth (High Priestess).

In a property question, **a structured routine, discipline, convention, tradition, learning, teaching or mentoring** may be the reason behind a particular rental or purchase.

Health and Well-being

This Hierophant reflects the **holistic (holy) trinity of health and well-being: what's good for the soul or spirit is inextricably good for the mind and body.**

This archetype can be **a person, group or organization who counsels, guides or helps others to make peace with their circumstances in times of stress, ill-health, depression or addiction** (Temperance). They can also represent **the peace, calm, harmony and stillness that come from a visit to a remote location** (Hermit, 6S), **sanctuary, retreat or rehabilitation centre, or simply taking regular quiet time out to meditate or contemplate** (4S).

The Hierophant adheres closely to **disciplined eating, drinking and exercise routines, using only tried and tested methods, medicines or treatments.** Unless influenced by unconventional cards (Fool, Magician, High Priestess), this archetype, who may be a medical professional themselves, **can perhaps stick a bit too closely to institutional advice.**

6 THE LOVERS VI

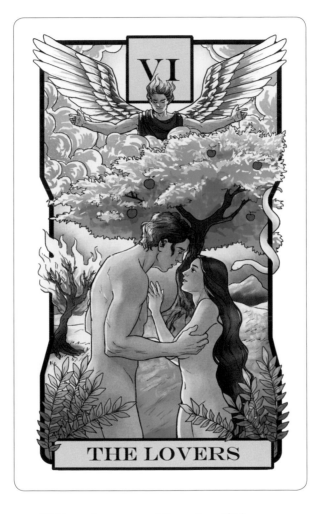

THE LOVERS

'If I have become a philosopher, if I have so
keenly sought this fame for which I'm still waiting,
it's all been to seduce women basically.'

JEAN-PAUL SARTRE

Personification – Psychology

As much of the Lovers' **emotional validation (Moon) is sought via their ability to attract lovers,** partners, friends, fans and admirers (Sun, 3C), this archetype indicates the potential for suffering (Tower, Moon) from any uncertain or insecure emotional attachments (Moon) that compromise self-esteem (9S).

The Lovers can indicate a major form of distraction, as their desirous or amorous frame of mind is too easily seduced (Devil) by new ideas, actions, emotions, environments or individuals (Aces).

As the metaphor of the Garden of Eden suggests, this archetype is often **unwilling to face or engage with unpleasant realities or hard truths (2S). New Lovers often view life through a rose-tinted prism, 'sugar-coating' or 'glossing over' the truth, or the consequences of eating a 'forbidden fruit'.**

However, this archetype also denotes **a higher voice of reason or wisdom, either an internal or external guiding voice, interceding with a strong message or advice.** The angel depicted in the Lovers cautions us that **placing too much importance on material or physical pleasures and even the outer appearances of objects or people (Empress) can be at the expense of our greater happiness and well-being.**

By releasing endorphins in the brain, pleasuring the physical senses has an effect similar to alcohol or sugar consumption and **renders the higher mind inoperable and the lower mind at its least discerning. By allowing the lower, snaking ego mind to dominate our thinking, the particular brand of sensual inebriation depicted in this archetype can lead it to make some really painful mistakes (Fool).** When this card presents itself in a reading, it is likely to be a **time to heed any higher, angelic advice.**

The cards connected to the Lovers act as agents that **negotiate the way in which our appreciation, approval and love of something or someone is applied in our life.**

Spirituality and Philosophy

Unless flanked by superconscious or spiritually awakened cards (Magician, High Priestess, Hermit), **it is this archetype's undisciplined pursuit of 'forbidden fruit', i.e. pleasuring of the physical senses, that most frustrates, but doesn't wholly deny, their spiritual progress.** Suffice to say, this card often signifies that **a higher decision needs to be made, one that requires greater faithfulness to your core beliefs or spiritual values.**

Alongside their psycho-emotional attachment (Moon) to sensual entertainment, pleasure and indulgence, it's the Lovers' **ego desire for love, admiration or adoration (Sun) that proves to be their greatest spiritual obstacle.**

The Lovers is the absolute opposite of renunciation (Hermit), and for those on the spiritual path (High Priestess), **love relationships can be exquisitely sweet distractions.**

Cards of material hardship (Hermit, 5P) presented alongside the Lovers can lend spiritual grounding and realism to the archetype, which would otherwise **prioritize mundane physical, material (Empress) or emotional (Moon) comforts over and above sacred or divine matters.**

Sun Tzu once said, 'If the mind is willing, the flesh could go on and on without many things,' meaning **what can be an uncomfortable process of self-realization is attained only by the perpetuity of mind over matter (Strength).**

Personal Life

In a relationship reading, **this card signifies, in its most modest expression (Temperance), the amorous attentions of another,** and in its most intense expression (Magician, Sun, Emperor, KW, QW, KnW), **a burning passion or fire in the loins that won't be extinguished** (1W).

It represents struggles with attraction (Empress), emotional attachment (Moon), desire, temptation, lust, carnal pleasure and sensual (Pentacles), intellectual (Swords), physical (Wands), emotional (Moon, Cups) love addictions or obsessions (Devil).

Unless the surrounding cards suggest otherwise, this archetype signifies **a relationship that is physically passionate but may lack substance.** The danger with this card is that **the physical aspect can wield too great a power or influence and make it difficult to see the truth of a situation.**

If a deep, sincere or emotionally connected and heart-centred commitment has been made (Empress, 1C, 2C, 10C, KC, QC), however, the Lovers can simply indicate that **the physical aspect of a partnership is good and healthy.** This is likely to be the **high point in your relationship in terms of attraction, romance, bonding, closeness, intimacy, connection, sex and physical intimacy.** Though, as is the law of nature, what goes up must come down, which will be the test of whether there is a real (1C, 2C) or imagined (Moon, 7C) heart connection.

This will be the moment our conscience, our higher voice of wisdom, intervenes and assists in a significant decision about a relationship or romantic pairing, helping us decide whether or not to take things to the next level (KC, QC, 2C, 4W) or call them off completely (Death, Tower, 5C, 3S).

The Lovers archetype can also represent emotionally sweet-natured individuals or those who suffer from regular sugar-crash-type love-withdrawal symptoms when each high or spike of psycho-sensual pleasuring begins to wane or fade (Moon). As a result, they often attract relationships that are co-dependent, emotionally, sensually or self-indulgent, and whose foundations are built solely on the saccharine pleasures of life and the sharing of hidden pleasure addictions (Moon, Devil). Pleasure-seeking and sensual gratification then become the psycho-emotional bedrock in a partnership, unless the individual benefits from self-discipline and regulation (Hermit, Hierophant).

The presence of this card can denote a range of problems that need addressing in an existing relationship. Perhaps, in the beginning, everything seemed perfect, but now the initial bliss is waning and the cracks are starting to show (Tower, 3S).

It can also indicate the end of the initial peacekeeping (Temperance) stage of a physical relationship, when partners are excessively obliging to each other (6C) at the expense of their own true needs, dreams and wishes (2S). This is the moment when each person's individual masculine energy begins to reassert its own agenda and priorities (Aces, Emperor). Whether the relationship survives beyond this point depends on how disruptive, destructive and shocking (Tower) the emergence of each partner's true needs, values and beliefs (Sun, High Priestess) are to the established relationship dynamic.

This is the defining make-or-break moment, when a person 'comes up for air' (KS, QS): when they begin to see clearly, logically and rationally whether their partner's long-term goals, inclinations and character truly align with their own.

When the initial intensity and excitement of sensual pleasuring, outward beauty or magnetism (Empress, Sun) start to relax, a partner's attitude can gradually turn from 'us first' back to 'me first'. Such superficial relationships, built solely on the thrill of seduction (KnW, KnC), infatuation and lust (Devil), then begin to crumble (Tower) or even end completely (Death).

When flanked by materially abundant cards (Emperor, Empress, KP, QP, 10P), the Lovers can signify the attraction of a huge change in your living standards, lifestyle or values due to your choice of partner. However, **the challenge of the Lovers archetype is in seeing beyond the obvious physical or sensual attractions to determine if there are the necessary factors that make for a more committed, longstanding relationship** (2C, 10C).

This card usually expresses some **ambivalence about a partner or romantic situation** (2P), or represents those who are unwilling (2S) to make any final judgement call on the future of their relationship. **The heart may be saying one thing and the head another, with the latter continually overriding, bypassing, dodging** (2S) or remaining blissfully ignorant (Fool) of the more **serious commitment question** (Hanged Man).

This may be the **time to take some space (Hermit, 4S) from a Lover to try and regain your lost perspective (Hanged Man) by allowing the diverting powers of the physical aspect (1W) to naturally wane and subside (Moon).**

When influenced by transparency-seeking cards (High Priestess, Sun, Hermit, KS, QS), **a moment of honest introspection can help determine whether a relationship will remain mutually satisfying in the long term or whether it is only skin deep.**

Professional Life

The presence of this archetype in a work reading suggests **the superficial aspects of physical, material attraction or sensual delight (Empress)** are key to the success of a work project, product or service (KP, QP, 10P, 9P).

The Lovers' nature is **to attractively package** new concepts and ideas (1S) and ways of making money (1P), emotionally (1C) or dramatically (1W) engaging new clients, customers and consumers.

When this card appears, **your personal life outside work could be in some way interfering with your professional life** (5W), resulting in a boss or co-worker questioning (KS, QS) or testing your commitment to a job or project (9W).

The Lovers can considerably **'raise the stakes' at work if you engage in office affairs and flirtations,** with either a co-worker (Knights) or your superior (Emperor, Empress, Kings and Queens). **Trouble in a paradisiacal job situation,** akin to the expulsion from the Garden of Eden, could result from disregarding the consequences of **mixing work and pleasure. This is not a time to allow your animal drives and desires (Devil) to overcome your better judgement.**

This archetype, in general, represents **a time to heed any higher guidance pertaining to work matters. Any advisory messages, emails or verbal communications should be actioned immediately, rather than put off, overlooked or ignored.**

Property – Finances – Resources

Adhering to the Lovers' laws of attraction, positive and expansive thinking (World, Moon) can provide greater financial opportunity and abundance (Magician, 10P) when this card appears in a reading. However, unless flanked by cards of wealth and material abundance, caution (Temperance) should be applied in all your financial dealings, as this archetype can represent **superficial or over-inflated estimates and valuations. Your stocks, shares and investments may attract great interest,** but whether they will continue to do so depends on the surrounding and outcome cards.

Under the influence of this archetype, **your emotional and/or ego desires can blind you (Moon, 2S) to any flaws and faults in a potential investment.**

By desiring, attracting or being attracted to sensual and material indulgences (KP, QP, 10P), you have huge potential for **thoughtless overspending (Fool) or whimsical purchases (PP)** under the influence of this archetype. The Lovers card makes you particularly prone to **buying items that make you appear more outwardly desirable and attractive, such as a grand property (Sun, 4W), flashy cars (Sun, Chariot) or beautifying clothing, accessories and cosmetics (Empress).**

Under the Lovers' influence, you may also make **a very attractive or desirable purchase, such as a 'des res' property, but unless cards are present to suggest otherwise, it may not be a logical (KS, QS), pragmatic or practical choice (KP, QP).**

Health and Well-being

The aforementioned Chinese strategist Sun Tzu once said, 'Do not swallow the bait offered by the enemy' – an interesting idea when we consider that our closest and most threatening enemy is our own lower mind and the bait its unconstructive, degenerate chattering (Devil, Moon). As such, the Lovers reminds us to pay greater attention to our inner dialogue. Similarly, the Lovers depicts **two diametrically opposing voices: the snake, symbolic of the lower, unrefined ego's (Devil) advice – to give in to physical desires – versus the higher, civilized angelic mind (Temperance) offering a lifeline.**

When their self-esteem is low or has taken a battering (Moon, 9S), this archetype indicates a preferred method of self-soothing via material or physical indulgences and sensory pleasures such as luxury, sweet or indulgent food and drink, perfumes, sex, massage or retail therapy – the problem being that the Lovers' sense of love, safety and security is then wholly dependent on them having obtained their sensual or material fix.

However, by realizing (Sun) and strengthening their inner resolve (Strength), this archetype can learn to fight (7W) and triumph over (Chariot, 6W) their **psycho-sensual dependencies.**

7 THE CHARIOT VII

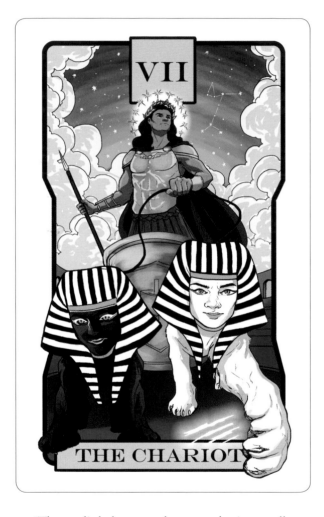

'The credit belongs to the man who is actually
in the arena, whose face is marred by dust
and sweat and blood.'
THEODORE ROOSEVELT

Personification – Psychology

Unless the **outstanding drive, focus, determination and endurance** of this archetype are in some way compromised by surrounding cards, the Chariot's **bold, brave, confident, daring, optimistic, assertive, attentive, self-assured, charged and ready-for-anything, do-or-die, no-mountain-is-too-high** approach **allows them to meet any challenge, opposition or competition head on, with victorious results (6W).**

As a **fighting spirit and competitive or challenging character (5W)**, the Chariot archetype, which **seeks victory in all things, only plays to win.** Being a **highly ambitious, 'going for gold', high-stakes risk-taker,** they are a physical, mental, emotional or spiritual force to be reckoned with. **Primed only for success, they are combative and aggressive in the pursuit of their wants, needs and goals,** always striving to exceed their own and others' expectations.

In addition to being **a winning spirit, they are driven by the passionate pursuit of a goal or cause,** something that gives their life meaning and purpose. **They know exactly what they want, and go for it by adopting a formidable strength of resolve and not stopping for any reason.** Unless flanked by impedimental cards (Hanged Man, 9W, 2S, 8S, 9S, 4P, 4C), **nothing can hold them back.**

They are drawn to all forms of **forward movement, progression or advancement.** Unless particular cards orient their trajectory towards matters of the past (Moon, 6C), **they rarely look back or behind them.**

As proponents of **swift and propulsive movement, they are exceptionally strong in overcoming emotional difficulties (Moon, 9S, 5C). They don't stop to question** or allow themselves to be caught up in the apathy (4C), doubt, confusion (Moon,

9S), resistance (9W), overthinking, over-analysing (8S), worry and anxiety (9S) that result in complete inertia (8S). Instead, **they quickly accept and adapt, surfing the arrhythmic and undulating happenstances of life.**

Pertaining to the Law of Attraction manifesting abundance or success, the tarot's warrior archetype epitomizes the idea that to 'win the day' you must jettison all doubt, hesitation and delay.

Aside from their great pace, flexibility of mind (KnS) and ever-ready presence (KnW), the Chariot's great successes can be attributed to **their uncanny ability to incorporate other perspectives into their own way of thinking and to reconcile diametrically different, opposing or contrasting views, be they internalized or drawn from external sources.**

Spirituality and Philosophy

This is an archetype **powered by their cosmic or divinely aligned connection to the higher guiding principle, also known as the complete and utter acceptance of what is, was and will be.**

They epitomize the idea of **peak-performing consciousness or spiritual fitness,** which comes from knowing how to best apply themselves in the world. This is discussed in the ancient Indian wisdom text the *Dhammapada* VIII, which states, **'The greatest of warriors is one who conquers the Self'** (Sun). The Chariot therefore represents the greatest of personal victories, **the winning of the raging internal battle (Moon, 5W)** between the mundane and spiritually oriented mind.

The Charioteer's battle is won via the diametrically opposed faction of the self, **the primitive, shadow, animal or ego aspect, being conquered, subdued and reintegrated with the higher, guiding principles of the civilized, humane mind (Temperance). When the conscious and shadow aspects of the psyche are fully** reconciled in this way, our free will is once again aligned with the will of the divine (Star).

The spiritual success of the Chariot is in **redirecting and fusing those opposing tensions** instead of allowing them to pull us this way and that. The lower ego mind pulls us one way, back towards ignorance and mundane concerns, and the higher mind pulls us another, towards the purely conscious source of en-lightenment from whence we originally came (Star, Sun). **Only when the wayward, destabilizing, unbalancing, ungrounded impulses of our old ego-conditioning cease to pull us off-centre can we find true peace of mind (Temperance).**

The Chariot is the antithesis of the stubborn, blinkered-old-mule mind (2S, 8S) attached to a flour grindstone or olive press, moving like the mundanely focused and circuitous ego mind in tight, constrictive, self-defeating circles (5S). When all aspects of the shadow self are fully integrated and reconciled, the psyche's driving forces can move more freely and efficiently, in a straight-forward rather than convoluted manner, from A to B, rather than A to B via P-A-I-N and S-U-F-F-E-R-I-N-G.

Though such mental theatrics or dramatic convolutions of thought (Devil) make for diverting stuff in the entertainment industry, **such diversions can be avoided when we progress on our personal and spiritual journey.** The beauty of the Chariot is in our sobering mentality, which moves us on from the intoxicating narratives we tell ourselves, be they ego-poking or stroking.

Based on the great insight of William Shakespeare, who stated in his play *As You Like It* that 'All the world's a stage, And all the men and women merely players,' we may argue that such dramatic convolutions are the purpose of life itself, and perhaps the more, the better, for what is life but a relentless series of instructive and improving experiences (Hierophant)? But far from messing with the divinely inspired blueprints of our lives

(Star), the progressive Chariot helps us integrate the lessons with greater speed and efficiency, rather than avoid them altogether. The Charioteer's spiritual success is in their ever-faithful and expansive vision (World). As nineteenth-century British philosopher James Allen wrote, 'A man can only rise, conquer, and achieve by lifting up his thoughts [Sun, Moon].'

Personal Life

In a relationship reading, the Chariot archetype is often favoured over any other competitor in a love match, either winning the battle for someone's affections or themselves being won over by another.

The Chariot also represents the successful healing of emotional battle wounds and scars, or the reconciling of polarized differences with a partner or polarized thoughts within yourself regarding a relationship so it can move forward.

Due to their fighting spirit, this archetype will make a huge effort to see a relationship through hard times (Tower, 5W). However, being the archetypal warrior, they often have difficulty letting their emotional guard down or showing their vulnerability (Moon, 9W). They may be more be interested in winning an argument than in resolving it amicably (5S).

They are the archetype most likely to use any means necessary to win the object of their desire – wealth and property (KP, QP), charisma, public profile or status (QW, KW) and/or intellect and knowledge (KS, QS) – and to be seeking a trophy wife or husband (9C).

Due to their 'winner takes all' attitude, the Chariot is also the archetype most prone to boundary issues in relationships, and can display a particular disregard for or inability to respect another's feelings if they try to block or impede (7W, 9W) their heated pursuit (1W). They are **likely to continue pursuing a potential mate (KnC, KnW)** irrespective of even the strongest signals that their desired object is not interested in them (2S, 7W, 4C).

The Chariot thrives on challenge, and their relationships can be initially intense and enthusiastic, but also, like the archetypal warrior, short-lived (3S, 5S, 5C). Once the object of their pursuit has been obtained and conquered, they lose their challenge value and subsequently the Charioteer's interest.

Yet, as the archetype of **self-preservation**, the Chariot's presence in a reading is a strong indication that a battle to honour and preserve the wants, needs and values of your true, core self in a relationship has been successfully fought and won.

Professional Life

The great success of this archetype ultimately springs from their **open, adventurous, exploratory or outwardly bound character and mentality**. It can indicate **the successful exploration of different work options, branching out, being headhunted and completely changing jobs or career trajectories (Wheel of Fortune), perhaps to work abroad (World, KnW)**. However, this **access all areas** archetype must be mindful not to encroach too much on someone else's territory, ideas, projects and job, especially via micro-managing (Emperor, 4P).

The Chariot's personality and modus operandi lend themselves well to any career where **the crossing of international or internal boundaries, barriers and borders is fundamental to success**. The Chariot energy is of paramount importance to the modern globalized world economy (World), **where, in a sense, everyone works for the greater good of all and interconnected business knows no boundaries (Star, 3W)**.

The Chariot **absorbs a great deal from other cultures and often welcomes the intervention of foreign powers or influences.** Hence they can achieve particularly great things when reconciling cultural differences of opinion in the work environment so that everyone goes forward together, in the same direction.

Property – Finances – Resources

If they so choose, the Chariot's **peak performance or outreaching efforts** can draw much public attention (Sun, World); under the influence of this archetype, any **outward-bound PR and marketing campaigns** can really pay off (World, 9P, 10P).

If you are looking for funding, the Charioteer can indicate **internationally sourced finances or resources** (World). They often make **impressive gains through their quick and efficient use of funds or get lucky breaks in high-risk ventures and investments (Strength).**

Financial failure is not an option for this archetype; being conditioned for only the greatest success, they win the day or land that big contract, client, campaign or project (6W) via sheer boldness, courage or bravado.

Unless flanked by compassionate or altruistic cards, **making gains from the downfall or misfortunes of others** can be the result of this **individualistic** archetype appearing in a reading. However, **if they are 'riding under another's banner', the Chariot's 'winner takes all' prize money can be directed** into more charitable (6P), equitable (Justice, Temperance), shared (3P, 3W, 3C) or mutually beneficial (2C, 2W) interests.

Health and Well-being

The many battles they have fought and won in the external world often mirror their own internal struggles (5W), which, if handled with self-conscious awareness (Sun), can lead to great inner and outer world mastery (Magician, World).

The presence of the Chariot in a reading, with their reconciled psychological aspects, epitomizes the battle strategy of Chinese philosopher Sun Tzu: 'If you know the enemy and know yourself, you need not fear the result of a hundred battles. If you know yourself but not the enemy, for every victory gained, you will also suffer a defeat. If you know neither the enemy nor yourself, you will succumb in every battle.'

Fortunately, due to the Chariot's fighting-fit, survivalist consciousness, they are able to show great warrior-like strength, endurance, flexibility and agility in combating all forms of sickness and disease.

8 STRENGTH VIII

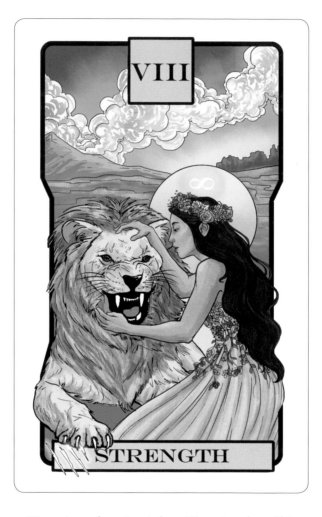

'Knowing others is wisdom. Knowing the self is
enlightenment. Mastering others requires force.
Mastering the self requires strength.'

LAO TZU

Personification – Psychology

Under the influence of this archetype, lust, arrogance and hubris or superiority complexes are understood and subdued by **humility, grace, elegance, loveliness, beauty, charm, decency, leniency, kindness, charity, compassion, sympathy, mercy and benevolence.**

The Strength principle protects the psyche (Moon) from its own and others' unintegrated wild, feral or animal drives, such as stealing (Devil, 7S), wounding (3S) and psychical debasement or attack impulses (Devil, Moon, 5W). It strengthens **graceful, civilized human impulses and instincts (Temperance)**, especially when they are threatened. It does this not by killing our wild animal aspects, for it exemplifies **the key Buddhist principle of non-violence towards ourselves and others,** but via **deep self-realization, taming, integrating and appropriating their power and strength for higher purposes.**

In becoming better friends with our whole selves and **befriending our 'inner beast',** we can pacify and vanquish our savage, feral, wild or predatory impulses and unwholesome emotions such as pride, arrogance and conceit. By allowing our higher mind to **captivate our wayward or animalistic 'monkey mind', we can induce ever-higher levels of conscious awareness (High Priestess, Magician)** and cease to be driven by devolved, mundane or base pursuits and interests.

Our archetypal Strength aspect is **powered by the facing of our fears – the repressed aspects of our self that we find most abhorrent or frightening.** Evoking the energy of this archetype can **subjugate and control any such fear-based thoughts (9S) or inhibitions (8S)** that may be holding us back from living a freer (Fool, Chariot), fuller and more fulfilled life (World).

When we work towards **integrating rather than forcefully rejecting, repressing, ignoring, disrespecting or over-**

intellectualizing our raw, wild, natural, instinctual, animalistic urges and behaviour, we avoid the fierce ego-snapback that comes from what Sun Tzu describes as pushing 'a desperate foe too hard'.

If the Strength archetype falls under a shadow influence (Devil), their intention to exert a positive influence over others can potentially become convoluted, resulting in **patronizing or condescending words or behaviour and considering all those who don't subscribe to their highly civilized behavioural ideals as inferior or beneath them.**

This archetype's ability to **maintain their composure at all times, their 'grace under fire', can also be a double-edged sword (1S), when fire really is the most pure and effective response.**

However, the most positive expression of this archetype is in **overcoming pride, conceit, vanity, ego and superiority to help bolster self-respect, esteem and regard, which then helps them recognize, reinforce and strengthen these personally fortifying forces in others.**

Spirituality and Philosophy

Strength's archetypical inner fortitude is not found in a physical or verbal show of strength or reacting aggressively to the affronting behaviour of others, but, conversely, in **holding back the urge to fight.** This archetype overcomes fears and apprehensions by **relinquishing power and control and accepting or allowing things to be as they are.**

So the Strength archetype doesn't 'fight fire with fire', but, via their higher, intuitive strength of mind (KS, QS, KnS), they avoid the battle altogether. This card exemplifies Sun Tzu's approach to contentious situations: 'Supreme excellence consists of breaking the enemy's resistance without fighting.'

Thus true inner Strength is **staying cool, calm, collected, meek, mild, unassuming, respectful, humble, patient and gentle. Keeping your head when everyone else is losing theirs.** As the Bible cautions, **'Blessed are the meek, for they will inherit the Earth.'** Considering when it was written, it is likely that this is a light reminder of the Strength archetype's staunchly non-violent and thus self-preserving continuity.

Personal Life

The Strength archetype can engender greater cooperation and balance in a relationship (2C) via their **infinite patience, understanding, peacemaking, soothing, comforting, calming, conciliation, placation, easing and appeasing.**

Characterized by **taking a softer approach**, especially when the other partner expresses the opposite behaviour, this archetype **maintains a peaceful, kind, loving, caring, close, considerate, harmonious, gentle, patient and forbearing ambience within a relationship.** Thus the Strength archetype signifies a transformative relationship, where **we grow into the best possible version of ourselves. When Strength is present, our needs are met and accommodated by others, not through forceful expectations or demands, but because they are negotiated gently and harmoniously.**

When this archetype knows things are finally over (Judgement, Death), or a partner is cheating or lying to them (Devil), they **simply gracefully detach from them with the least possible fuss and resistance (Temperance). As Sun Tzu advised, 'The wise warrior avoids the battle.'**

Indeed, the inner Strength of this archetype is wholly reliant on **letting our guard down in a relationship, emotional exposing ourselves or showing our vulnerability and strengthening the** bond of intimacy with another person by trusting our heart is safe in their hands. In overcoming the fear of rejection and squarely facing the possibility of grief and disappointment, we open ourselves up to the strongest possible love connection.

In a personal reading, the virtuous temperament of this archetype, rising above its animal drives and instincts, can reflect a higher-minded decision to resist sleeping with a partner or indulging the physically needy aspect of our own character.

Professional Life

This is the archetype of calm, collected, civilized and higher-minded work meetings, negotiations, discussions and conversations. Strength tends also to bring a civilized or sophisticated look, edge or outcome to creative processes, projects, work or business.

Success comes from taking a gentle, subtle, passive, mutually supportive, cooperative, respectful and feminine approach to work issues, rather than an aggressive, competitive, masculine one. The Strength archetype works well and efficiently for the higher good of all.

When this card appears, the initial raw hunger for a career or project, the desire to be a professional, to be a winner (Emperor), may be somewhat reduced. Regardless, due to their 'feel the fear and do it anyway' attitude, the Strength archetype thrives in risky business ventures and environments where financial speculations are being made on a daily basis. They see great results when they allow themselves to be vulnerable, perhaps by courageously risking their reputation in making public (Sun, 8W) a new and untested project or product (1W, 1P).

The key to this archetype's success when attending a professional test, trial or interview is in their refined and transparent 'guard down' demeanour, which allows them to be seen as fearless in their vulnerability.

Property – Finances – Resources

Strength passively allows material abundance to come to them (Hanged Man), rather than actively, forcefully or aggressively 'chasing the money'. Applying their refined, domestic or higher-minded principles, they manage to quietly curb the wilder ego impulse to overspend or indulge in flashy or expensive items, and tend, generally, to avoid frivolous purchases or base financial decisions. Their purchases and investments are, instead, usually made only after **taking the most highly informed advice from the most refined sources.**

Paradoxically, as a card of speculation, the Strength archetype is then prone to using **this higher guidance to play big in risky financial ventures (Wheel of Fortune).** Yet, due to their centred approach, their speculative gambles can pay off handsomely (Sun, 10P).

Health and Well-being

When flanked by positively toned cards, the Strength archetype symbolizes **robust health and physical fortitude, recovery from sickness and restoring strength to a weakened or compromised immune system.**

It also symbolizes **the power to overcome anything** mentally (KS, QS, 1S), emotionally (KC, QC, 1C), energetically (KW, QW, 1W) or materially (KP, QP, 1P), and so can represent the remission, subduing or controlling of a previously raging illness.

Strength copes successfully with health imbalances, either by following higher counsel and advice or by adopting a passive, non-aggressive or non-violent approach.

This card often denotes a period of **self-healing, implemented via the power of our own mind to calm our nerves and anxieties. This is likely to be a time to successfully vanquish any natural physical urges to overindulge, such as binge-eating, drinking or drug-taking.**

However, **those whose natural animal impulses and emotions have been blocked, repressed or insufficiently processed and released can endure physical health problems, which will be the human body's way of showing psychological dis-ease.**

The modern resurgence and continued popularity of the Second World War poster produced by the British government depicting the royal emblem of the crown with the slogan **'Keep calm and carry on'** epitomizes the sometimes **repressive gracefulness of this archetype, which often then finds a 'more civilized' way to purge their internalized emotional pain, anger and frustration.** In the documentary *In Her Own Words*, the late Diana, Princess of Wales, spoke in such terms of the infidelity of her husband and her bulimia: **'I was rejected, I didn't think I was good enough for the family, so I took it out on myself . . . I decided to do the more discreet thing . . . and it always felt better after I'd been sick to get rid of the anger.'**

In general, unless flanked by publicity- or attention-seeking cards (Sun, KW, QW, KnW), this archetype **tends towards the quiet and graceful receiving of health-related news.** The inner strength and fortitude they cultivate may also lead them to **play down an illness in order to avoid drawing attention to them- selves or being fussed over.** Friends and family should remain conscious of this, for more than any other, **this archetype tends towards suffering in silence.**

9 THE HERMIT IX

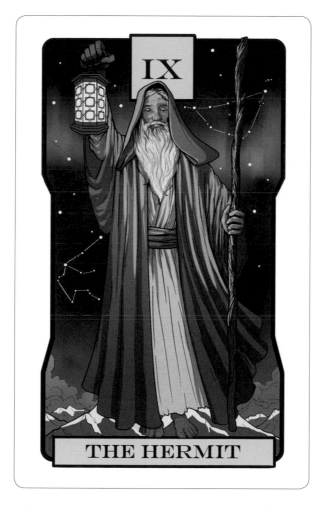

'Great minds discuss ideas; average minds discuss
events; small minds discuss people.'
ELEANOR ROOSEVELT

Personification – Psychology

This archetype signifies a period of clearing your life and mind of all their mundane and trivial preoccupations to make a consistent and permanent space for higher-level thoughts – the key to independent survival, via a grounded sense of self-reliance or invaluable faith in your inner intelligence, strength and resources. For instance, learning how to self-parent (Moon), and subsequently bettering your parenting or caretaking skills in the process, can fill or inspire those under the influence of this archetype with a new confidence in their own self-sufficiency and unique or individual abilities (3P).

The Hermit's mentality (1S) of mature realism and seriousness is often the result of a significant disappointment or failed expectations (Tower, Death, 3S, 5C, 5P, 5S), the higher purpose being that the old, ineffectual identity must be released (Death, Tower, 10S) so that a new, mature self can emerge (Star, Aces). However, this archetype's new-found wisdom can sometimes feel sacrificial (Hanged Man) or particularly hard-won (5S, 5W, 5C, 5P).

The Hermit is seriously engaged in integrating unwieldy ego forces, forces that prevent self-realization by keeping the mind anchored in mundane matters rather than focused on more spiritual concerns, and through concerning themselves solely with their interior thoughts, they force their own self-isolation. This isolation, and the closing off of the sense organs, impede the access of all the besieging exterior forces that would otherwise engage the mundanely occupied mind. So the advice of Sun Tzu to 'Be where your enemy is not' is the key philosophy of the Hermit archetype, whose enlightenment is made possible by isolating themselves from the external influences that stroke the ego.

Put another way, in the words of A. A. Milne, creator of Winnie the Pooh, bear of 'little brain' with a largely **philosophical sacred outlook**, 'The third-rate mind is only happy when it is thinking with the majority. The second-rate mind is only happy when it is thinking with the minority. The first-rate mind is only happy when it is thinking.' Thus it is **the maturely self-reliant, direct, first-hand subjectively experiencing mind of the Hermit, turned inward towards the sacred, that finds true contentment and happiness**.

Whether we attain the fullest possible state of inner conscious awareness or self-realization is largely dependent on contemplative hermitage periods. **Periods of isolation** undertaken by choice, rather than involuntarily, will **disable any ego resistance and turn any suffering experienced into an opportunity for personal and spiritual development.**

When we reach the peak of a personal or spiritual phase of growth, it can be that irreconcilable conflict between our newly emerging psyche and its old external support network (Moon, Death, 5W) leads to **a feeling of isolation and loneliness.** If our shadow aspect (Devil) is the root cause of this isolation, then **entering into a dialogue with this separatist energy, ugly though it may be, provides a great opportunity to become self-realized, healed and happy.** Thus the human aspects that are seen as socially isolating actually have the most crucial role to play in our overall personal and spiritual development (Wheel of Fortune), and so should be savoured and valued rather than feared and resisted.

By practising complete non-attachment to mundane or material existence, the Hermit is mostly drawn to plain, simple, ordinary, ascetic, sober, austere, unadorned, undecorated, unembellished, sparse, abstinent, frugal, severe, humble and penitent ways of life.

Because their sense of self-satisfaction, fun, play or self-expression (Sun), security, protection and comfort (Moon) isn't

derived from mundane socializing or external distractions and sensory pleasures, their life can look outwardly dry or sober. Yet their inner world is abundantly rich and engaging.

Spirituality and Philosophy

The Hermit archetype suggests that right now a certain amount of hardship is necessary to attain the highest level of spiritual realization. Those seeking deeper drawn spiritual insight may have to endure hardship and renunciation while demonstrating the moral, ethical and disciplined approach key to furthering the spiritual maturation process.

By rejecting external sensory pleasures, entertainments and diversions, the Hermit sharpens (1S) their interior senses. For this archetype, subtle and subjective truth takes precedence over any mass objective consensus of 'reality'. As Carl Jung explained in *Memories, Dreams, Reflections*, 'The dream is outside; the reality is inside.'

The Hermit's subjective interiority augments their under-standing of their own and others' psychological and emotional projections (7C, Moon), and so augments 'reality' rather than being at the expense of it, as modern reductionist science would have us believe.

The Hermit's period of isolation also allows for a longer and deeper mental purification (Sun, Moon), whereby the ego's immature 'my way' decision-making processes can mature into more appropriate and inclusive responses and directives.

It is only via the Hermit's inclination to look inward, to become independently self-realized, that the benefits of our interior intelligence can be properly recognized and understood.

Personal Life

Despite having satisfying personal relationships, the Hermit archetype is very comfortable alone and even **values their solitude.** As a wisdom-seeker, they know that what your mind can conjure up when you are alone is often far more remarkable than what it produces when it is preoccupied with other people.

As such, rather than having a multitude of superficial friends or acquaintances, **the Hermit usually only puts energy into a few close relationships.** This makes meeting romantic partners more challenging, but their current life focus, whether they are conscious of it or not, is on personal development anyway.

Therefore, the presence of this archetype in a reading usually signifies a period of **needing to be on your own, whether by remaining single or taking a break from an existing relationship.** You realize that **the answers you seek are within you, and so you go your own way.**

Undergoing this process while remaining in a partnership can lead to a more **mature and independent (Hermit), rather than co-dependent (Lovers, Moon), way of relating (2C, 10C),** though this archetype's feelings aren't any less committed or sincere. Instead, **as a by-product of their own self-love, respect and esteem, their feelings are often more authentic and loving.**

Jetsunma Tenzin Palmo, the British Tibetan nun who went to live in an isolated cave in the Himalayas, spoke of the underlying principle of the Hermit's **fearless feeling** when she said, 'People, especially family, get upset if you are not attached to them, but that's only because we confuse love and attachment all the time.'

Like a monk, priest, nun or medieval anchorite who wishes above all else to **pursue their spiritual life goals and enter into an ever-deeper relationship with the divine, the Hermit can** indicate a resistance to secular relationships, marriage, procreation and childbirth (High Priestess, Hierophant, 1S, 2S, QS, KS). When paired with cards that are similarly focused on spiritual objectives (KS, QS, High Priestess, Hierophant), it may indicate a complete detachment from material or physical desires and all the attachments that are bound up with them (Strength).

Thus this card in a romance or relationship reading indicates that a higher purpose is taking priority over your personal life. This is a huge opportunity to strengthen your character or personal resolve and to master the art of self-reliance, self-care and psychological independence, so you can independently tackle anything life throws at you in the future.

This stage in your personal development can really upset the balance of any pre-existing relationships. However, a wholly conscious relationship, where the partners rely on their interior intelligence rather than the exterior validation of the other person, can survive and even thrive after such a change in the relating dynamic.

Professional Life

The Hermit archetype can symbolize solitary or private work, studies, interests, hobbies and pastimes, self-employment, self-orientated work and the proverbial one-man band. This card indicates working from home, in an isolated setting, laying low, keeping your head down, maintaining a low profile or keeping your own counsel at work.

This archetype also represents a time of disengaging from the outside world and already established or popular culture, and looking solely within for your inspiration and answers. Its aversion to the mainstream, to company or establishment policy, often results in **independent or separatist actions and movements. Doing things on their own terms, the Hermit may alienate** others but ensure their own positive personal development results in the long term.

Such is the **self-reliant nature** of this archetype that **their greatest wisdom doesn't come vicariously through the experience of others, but instead is entirely self-realized (Hierophant).**

When we have many options before us (7C) and aren't sure which path to take (Moon), the Hermit can symbolize taking time out for **contemplative soul-searching, perhaps a gap year abroad (Chariot) before embarking on a serious course of study.**

After spending twelve years in her Himalayan hermitage, Jetsunma Tenzin Palmo spoke of the longer-term benefits of **giving ourselves time and space to grow,** when she advised, '"Being" is **often better than "doing" and taking time out to be still and think is often a better investment for future productivity than cramming every waking moment with feverish activity.'**

To the modern objective observer, it may seem that the isolation of the Hermit is a form of inactivity, procrastination or work-shyness, and yet just **simply being with ourselves, alone, is so much harder than being in the company of others, who form the perfect outward distraction – a noisy distraction that often drowns out the wise and knowing words of our true, intuitive inner voice.** Thus time alone is the only way to find our true selves and initiate a deeply fulfilling self-realized (Magician, High Priestess) and self-actualized (World) existence.

When we cease to actively seek any attention, praise or recognition for our work or study efforts, we cultivate a humble core security and strengthen our interior intelligence. Such spiritually constructive periods of isolation, no matter how long they last, should be undertaken with a view to eventually sharing our unique contributions with the world (World).

Property – Finances – Resources

Being primarily orientated towards the immaterial, spiritual or sacred, the Hermit may work towards **reducing their physical or material concerns**, finding more pleasure in relinquishing than making material acquisitions. Thus this card can represent a time of **letting go of material attachments or financial obligations.**

This archetype can also indicate a **self-made man or woman who knows how to draw on their own wellspring of inner resources.**

By virtue of their independent streak, this archetype may be drawn to living self-sustainably and off-grid, or perhaps in a private, secluded, isolated, remote, sequestered, cloistered location or retreat.

Often this card coincides with **a test, to see if we can go it alone and survive on our own terms, and can, therefore, indicate the time is nigh for leaving home or living on our own.**

Health and Well-being

The Hermit can take **great solace from any period of isolation,** where, according to Jetsunma Tenzin Palmo, '**The answer lies within ourselves. If we can't find peace and happiness there, it's not going to come from the outside.**' The Hermit relishes these **quieter moments, seeing them as opportunities to grow and mature,** even when they are born of life's hardships, difficulties and challenges.

As nature intended, our growth, like that of flora and fauna, is a hidden, private, benighted and Hermit-like affair. This is why this archetype remains on the best possible terms with solitude.

The moment of the Hermit's greatest triumph (Chariot, 6W) comes when the comfort, protection and sustenance (Moon) usually provided by close friends and family cease or are restricted (3S, 5P, 5C). **This induces an uncomfortable (Moon) and intensified (10W) yet unparalleled period of maturization, emotional self-reliance and inner resourcefulness. By accessing their deepest internal wellspring (1C), the Hermit then finds a veritable fountain of self-care, love and nourishment (1C) ready and waiting.**

The Hermit isolation agenda thus helps instil the deep understanding that no persons or agencies outside yourself can match the support provided by your own inner healer, caretaker, protector, parent and anchor.

10 THE WHEEL OF FORTUNE X

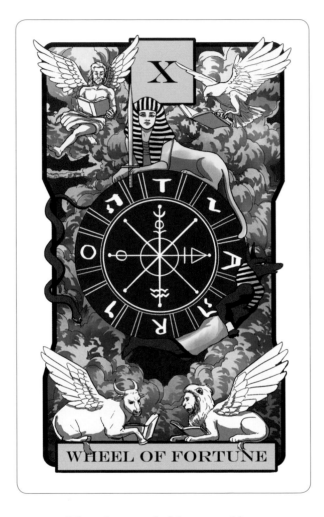

'There is no such thing as accident;
it is *fate* misnamed.'
NAPOLEON BONAPARTE

Personification – Psychology

When the Wheel of Fortune appears in a reading, an important event, situation or person will impact and change your outlook on life. This is **a major turning-point,** where anything is possible (Fool), **everything is in flux and great changes are afoot.** Be they internal or external, **predetermined, predestined, preordained forces of change** are working to reorient your life. Your fate is 'written in the stars' or 'in the lap of the gods': your **destiny is calling (Judgement).**

In light of the Old English etymology of 'fate' or similarly 'destiny', meaning 'that which comes, becomes, turns or turns into', we understand that nothing can be done to change a situation once the Wheel is in motion. The Wheel of Fortune is a card of inevitability, of **natural, unstoppable forces at work:** what goes up must come down, to rise up again. There is no avoiding it.

By riding, rather than reluctantly running to catch up with the Wheel of Life, you can, however, turn any situation to your advantage (Magician). Adopting a constantly open, agile mindset (Magician) will take you to **new places (Chariot)** and help you **move on from the past (Judgement).** The cards surrounding this archetype can express both the suffering that accompanies any **futile resistance to a major life change (Tower, Death, 3S, 9S, 10S, 5P, 5C)** or the clean speed and liberation of rolling with it (Fool, Chariot, World, KnS, 8W).

The outcome may be somewhat fixed, but the way you experience it is not. Treating any major change as disruptive, unwelcome or involuntary will only make you feel more insecure (Moon). 'Luck' is not simply the case of **fulfilling your destiny,** but also the result of your expectations and attitude (Moon); thus by **gracefully accepting each new era of your life, you will find fate will always smile upon you.**

The Wheel of Fortune helps you understand your personal and spiritual development cycles in terms of a series of contrasting positions. Rather than being feared and resisted, time spent down under the ever-moving Wheel should be savoured and valued as **crucial to growth and transformation**. For **the grand, destined, karmic luck, success and happiness** symbolized by the upward ascent of the Wheel are only made possible via a descending turn through difficulties, challenges and irritations.

When your will is **wholly aligned with the will of the divine and you take any major change it offers in your stride (Temperance)**, things can move forward at an exponential rate. When the path towards your life goals is internally cleared and clarified, no obstacle can stop your higher destiny from taking shape.

Spirituality and Philosophy

The Wheel of Fortune symbolizes the ups and downs of **human duality**, including but not limited to love (Sun) and hate (Devil), selflessness (Temperance) and self-absorption (4P), spirituality (High Priestess, Cups) and sense-perception (Lovers, Pentacles), disengagement (Hermit) and addiction (Devil), integrity (High Priestess, Swords) and distortion (Devil, 7C), admiration (Sun, Hierophant) and fanaticism (Devil, Sun), aspiration (World) and desire (Devil, 4P), firmness (Emperor) and vulnerability (5P, 5C, 9S), impartiality (Justice) and envy (Devil), bliss (Sun) and sorrow (5C, 3S), transcendence (Star, World) and mundanity (4P).

It also represents **our gradual release from the paralysing grip of fear and the intense experience of reawakening to the divine truth within ourselves**.

Anubis, the jackal-headed god on the ascending side of the Wheel, acquired his role as a guide to the ancient Egyptian underworld due to his **inherent duality**. Jackals appear active only in the transition times of sunrise and sunset and where the lush life of the Nile-fertilized land meets the unfertile desert, marking out both the time and place where dark and light, day and night meet. Each turn of the Wheel signifies **the dynamic tensions between these contrasting forces: the contrasting states of our human being.**

Human consciousness is cyclical, moving in and out, up and down, on its ultimate journey towards the fully awakened state. But with each upward turn of the Wheel, we become aware of the means of this **spiritual renewal.**

The fixed zodiac signs in each corner of the card guide the development of our higher awareness. Their fixed positions act as milestones on our journey to **more refined and elevated levels of spiritual awareness.**

The spinning motion of the Wheel symbolizes **the raising and refining of this awareness,** just like wheat is milled and ground down to flour via the many revolutions of a circling mule moving a grindstone. The Wheel of Fortune's alchemical milling motion gradually separates the imperishable golden kernel of the pure human spirit from its concealing ego husk.

So the Wheel speaks of a lifelong journey to **an ever more refined state of heart–mind equilibrium** via the acceptance, balancing and reconciliation of our dualistic and opposing forces of light and shadow (Justice, Temperance, Chariot). Only via such **spiritual refinement** can we ever truly know the divine state within all of us.

Personal Life

The Wheel of Fortune in a relationship reading symbolizes **a fixed or definite change that is unavoidable**. This could be a significant upturn in your relationship status, perhaps an engagement or marriage (2C, 3C, 4W), having a child or deciding to start a family (Aces, Pages), or **a major relationship or marriage ending (Justice, Death, Tower)**.

This archetype can also signify a **cyclical, unsettled** partnership (Lovers), where, as the ancient Greek philosopher Heraclitus once said, '**Change is the only constant**' (Moon). So if you decide to remain in such a relationship, it will serve you best to have no expectations, or **expect the unexpected, in order to maintain calmness and clarity (Temperance) in the face of any major shifts and changes.**

If you are single, this card can signify the commencement of a significant relationship that is likely to **revolutionize your life.**

Professional Life

In saying, 'I'd rather have lucky generals than good ones,' the French emperor Napoleon Bonaparte captured the essence of the Wheel of Fortune. For, when flanked by positively toned cards, this archetype signifies **unforeseen luck in work and business**. It can mean **a life-changing new job opportunity** or a prosperous start to a new business (Aces), a highly beneficial or advantageous situation and great revolutionary advances in your career.

New career orientations at this time can take you down a completely different path in life and you may be given far more responsibility (Emperor, Empress). The film *E.T.* began, according to director Steven Spielberg, with him trying to write a story about his parents' divorce, and, **as fate would have it,** that film launched his career. Interestingly, Spielberg also said, 'Casting sometimes is fate and destiny more than skill and talent, from a director's point of view,' which summarizes this archetype's fortuitous view of life.

This isn't to say skill and talent (3P) aren't important, simply that there is a right time and place for everyone to shine (Sun). When, where and how must be **in alignment with your clearest and most refined interests, as pertaining to divine will.** When something is truly meant to be, the circumstances of your life will magically transform (Magician) to make it so. This is not something you can plan or control, for the Wheel of Fortune will remain **ever unpredictable.** As soon as you think you have life figured out, you cease to grow and evolve, and that is when **the Wheel turns and the cycle of change begins once again.**

Property – Finances – Resources

The Wheel of Fortune can mark **a major change in your financial affairs,** either for the better or the worse, depending on the surrounding cards. If the surrounding cards are negative, the looming threat of a cut in funding or financial support may finally come to pass, meaning that you have to shut down a business or lose your job (Death). It may be that you have invested your money unwisely (Devil) and you now face much reduced circumstances or even bankruptcy as a consequence (Tower, 10S, 5P).

When supported by positively toned cards, however, the wheel is 'luck side' up, making **the odds more favourable.** During this period positively invested time or money may result in a major material manifestation (Magician). A well-judged risk or gamble (Strength) may have paid off, providing a life-changing amount of money, or you may make providential returns on your investments (Magician, Emperor, Empress, World, 9P, 10P) that set you firmly on the way to a new and more prosperous lifestyle. Making significant material investments, moving house, area or country (Chariot, World) are all possibilities when the Wheel of Fortune is on the turn.

With the presence of certain cards, an irreversible change in your financial circumstances may have already taken place (Judgement); if the Wheel has taken a downward turn, know that there is a higher reason behind this: your path to true contentment and happiness is paved not with material but spiritual riches.

Health and Well-being

The presence of the Wheel of Fortune in a health and well-being reading signifies that **change and motion** are what's needed: your life is being renewed, refreshed or revolutionized (Aces) after a long period of inertia or stagnation (Hanged Man, 8S).

This archetype signifies **all cyclical patterns of sickness and health (Moon), such as the push and pull, up and down cycles (2P)** of dizziness, motion sickness, restlessness, insomnia, menstruation, menopause (Moon), **conception, birth, new generations (Aces) and old age (Emperor, Hermit).**

The presence of this card can represent a life-changing illness or recovery from the same. As Marcus Aurelius once said, 'The universe is change, our life is what our thoughts make it.' Thus if life brings a great involuntary change, know you still have the choice to face it fearlessly (Strength).

11 JUSTICE XI

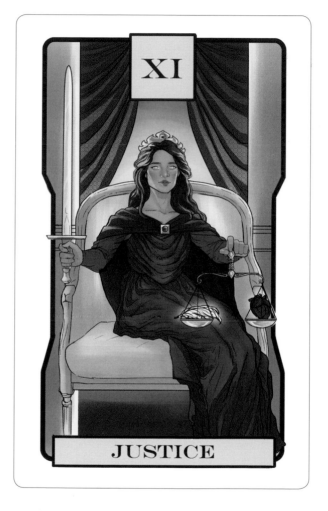

'The wheels of justice grind slow, but grind fine.'
SUN TZU

Personification – Psychology

Karma, or nature's law of cause and effect, ensures that what goes around comes around. You reap what you sow, or get your just deserts. Yet the 'jury', whether literal, social or divine, can remain out on a matter for some time (2S). However, when flanked by selfless, altruistic, harmony-seeking cards, Justice represents any environment where things have fallen out of balance or alignment but are **realigning, rebalancing and being put to rights (Temperance).**

Being primarily concerned with **moral geography,** the Justice archetype **presides over all iniquitous behaviour:** falsehood, cheating, theft, the destruction of property, violence, lying, fraud, sexual misconduct, self-deception, the pollution of land, water, your own or another's body and mind, etc. Only when we conduct ourselves in a morally irreprehensible way or **accept complete responsibility** for our negatively impacting words or actions can **the wisdom and maturity** of the Justice archetype be realized.

Justice symbolizes **a judicial or judge's mentality:** worldly (World), informed, astute, honest, fair-minded, balanced, equitable, impartial, independent, objective, nonaligned, open-minded, unbiased, dispassionate, neutral, detached, unprejudiced and redressing any perceived imbalances (KS, QS). This archetype, in **weighing both sides of the argument, sees the real truth of a matter and gets their facts straight** before making a final decision on what is right and just (Judgement). So this can indicate a time long past being given **the benefit of the doubt (Moon).**

When this archetype appears in a reading, you may be expending too much mental energy (Moon, 5S, 9S) on **mind-mapping an ever-growing inventory of others' offences.**

Whether it be the Justice of a large-scale political or military endeavour or a small-scale personal or domestic issue, you may be hosting **raging internal or external discussions about who or what is right or wrong (5W)**.

The overarching conviction that allows a person to believe they are 'right' is usually the result of previous direct experience, emotional trauma, education, social conditioning and upbringing. Justice's **upright Sword of Truth** can cut through **convictions that are the by-products of false or misleading thought patterns**. This archetype holds you to **ethical or moral codes of conduct and the laws of the land** set out for your own benefit and protection.

Justice also symbolizes the laws of nature, such as **like attracting like** and **the law of cause and effect,** by which the Justice archetype advises that what you put into a situation, you get back. Pertaining to this natural law, individuals who seek attention may attract highly visible or public (Sun) **judicial-type situations,** becoming the main spectacle in a newsworthy **court case** in which all hidden truths (High Priestess) are revealed and legal, social or moral justice is served for the greater good and higher learning of all concerned – 'all' meaning the wider world audience (Hanged Man).

Based on the law of cause and effect, when your actions are **true, pure and well-intentioned,** when the moment comes for you to be judged by any surrounding forces, you will be **shown to be right, vindicated, cleared of any wrongdoing or proved innocent (6W)**. The victory might be particularly sweet (Chariot, 9C, 6W) if you have suffered a major injustice at the hands of others (Devil).

Spirituality and Philosophy

The Justice archetype can be seen as a **balancing or reconciliation of heart and mind, or light and shadow energies, when the two have fallen out of alignment or become too polarized.** This is the inner, metaphysical working that creates and determines our experience of the physical world.

When this archetype appears in a reading, **forces are gathered around you to test and judge your spiritual progress.** They remind you to ask yourself, 'Am I following a path of truth, authenticity and justice, or rerouting away from it?'

Higher divine truth sustains the words, acts and deeds of those living in accordance with it, but undermines those who are not. The Justice archetype works with divine truth, **nourishing our higher, purer and untainted aspects.** So Justice also means recognizing and transforming the conditioned aspect of your mind so it realigns with **the truth of your divinely inspired and innately pure heart centre** (Magician). The extent to which your ego has fallen out of alignment with your heart centre is the extent to which you will experience **the sharp edge of Justice's sword. This Sword of Truth** (1S), like Justice's piercing gaze, **cuts through all mentally constructed falsehood** (7C). So Justice symbolizes the **external moral forces working on your spiritual interior, which subsequently carve your experience of external, material reality;** whether you feel the sharp edge of the Sword of Truth (1S) depends on how true you have been to yourself and others.

Understanding the world in these dualistic terms as a series of balancing contrasts or opposites in equilibrium, like heaven and Earth, good and bad, is to understand the human condition. **Justice is the rebalancing of the archetypal principles of polarity and opposition:** when a person's truth is weighed against that of their own heart. This is **the ultimate judgement of their spiritual progress,** for the heart symbolizes a person's pure spiritual essence, and a well-balanced mind–heart connection is one in which the forces of the psyche are as free as the spirit – free from mundane concerns.

Just as the Sword of Truth (1S) stands upright, so **the awkwardly embodied soul or spirit can also be 'straightened' out by upright behaviour.** Then the soul, having been **cut free from any wayward impulses,** can rest easy, **perfectly clear, pure, balanced and attuned to the heart-centralized position of truth, order and justice.**

Personal Life

The weighing of the heart against a feather symbolizes **the establishing of the right relationship with yourself and others. Untruths weigh heavy on the heart,** tipping relationships out of balance. **Making an honest declaration of your feelings and intentions,** whether they are good and true or not, will bring you into accordance with divine truth, order and justice. **By honouring the truth within yourself,** you can achieve a feather-light heart, perfectly centralized and balanced with the motivations of the mind.

Justice symbolizes **honouring your higher truth and defending it from the wayward opposing forces** that seek to make you blind to it, such as lust and physical obsession (Devil, Lovers). Thus **attaining equilibrium (Temperance)** between opposing mind-born and heart-born desires is fundamental to the ideal of **perfect truth, order and justice in a relationship.** So the critical question this card asks in a relationship reading is: **'Are the emotional forces of my psyche attuned to the deepest or purest wishes of my heart?'** If the answer is 'yes', your heart centre will be light like a feather, or en-lightened, the balance will be perfect and your love life will flow smoothly. If you are making choices in your life which are unaligned with the deepest wishes of your heart, the balance will be tipped, your heart will feel heavy, your love life will cease to flow and your emotions stagnate.

In a relationship reading, this archetype also symbolizes the truth coming out regarding an **injustice, unfairness, inequality or imbalance in a relationship** (High Priestess, KS, QS).

Justice sees and understands all sides and perspectives, and has an exceptional sense of integrity. It doesn't take another person's side in an argument just to appease, placate, pacify or conciliate them (Strength). Thus it could be that you are experiencing harsh but balanced and lawful treatment (KS, QS, KnS) from your chief nurturers or protectors (Empress, Emperor, Moon). Under opposing influences to the ideals of truth and justice (Devil), you may even be living under the constant **fear (Moon) of a reprisal or payback by a punitive or lawyer-like partner, friend or family member.**

This card suggests a legal aspect to a relationship, so marriage is in the offing when the surrounding cards are positive, and a divorce settlement, which could go either way depending on whether amicable or disagreeable cards are present, when they are not. By remaining **detached, impartial and independent in your judgement,** you could be viewed by a co-dependent partner as cold and distant. However, the guidance of this archetype, especially if you are tying up loose ends in your personal life (Death, Judgement), is to **stay centred, grounded and impartial in emotionally challenging situations.**

Professional Life

This archetype is often concerned with all forms of **alliances, agreements, deal-making, bargaining, trade, negotiations, brokerage, contracts (Temperance), equity and equality** for the purposes of shared or mutual interests (2C, 2W). This includes a business deal or contract being negotiated (1W, 2W, 3W), the offer of a permanent (9C, 10C) or temporary (2S, 8S, Moon) contract, or a foreign work visa (3W, KnW, World).

This archetype also represents a legal mentality that dots the 'i's and crosses the 't's in situations where paying attention to the details is key. It is the concurrent, conforming and concordant energy (KC, QC, KnC) that binds or breaks **all promises, agreements, arrangements, covenants, treaties, settlements, understandings, pacts, bonds, accords, unions (Temperance) and confidentiality agreements (High Priestess).**

Due to these **refined skills and abilities (3P)** in **diplomatic negotiations (Temperance)**, Justice therefore represents **the final resolution of conflict (6W)**, both internal (Moon) and external, such as a legal dispute (4W).

Property – Finances – Resources

In accounting or financial matters, this archetype symbolizes **the books being balanced** and any outstanding monies being paid, or adequate compensation for any losses or inconveniences.

Being the card of legal dealings, it covers **all contractual financial commitments**, like mortgages, loans or purchasing something on credit (6P). It also represents all forms of conveyancing, including the buying and selling of land and property (4W, 10P) or any valuable item that requires **official**

documentation to change the legal ownership, such as a vehicle (Chariot).

When this archetype appears, the advice is to attend to **the legal side of your business or financial affairs.** If you have kept things above board, the outcome will be financially favourable. If Justice is surrounded by negatively toned cards, however, you or your company may be facing **legal action,** so the only person who benefits will be the lawyers.

Health and Well-being

Applied to health and well-being, Justice can be enacted in a number of ways: through reaping the benefits of **a more balanced diet or exercise programme,** taking up a form of **exercise involving ordered, structured movements and balancing postures,** or treating others as you wish to be treated yourself. The latter can result in a marked improvement in your **mental and emotional balance, and so general happiness (Sun).** This, subsequently, attracts like-minded individuals, who have an equally positive effect on your life.

Conversely, you may be experiencing the **negative emotional or physiological results** of not attending to your health and well-being. You may be **reaping the consequences of bad habits** such as compulsions, obsessions or overindulgences (Devil, Moon) of drugs, alcohol, eating or physical pleasures (Lovers).

If you are not one to overindulge, it may be you need to let go of your **critical inner judge** telling you that you are not worthy. Similarly, **an imbalanced, heavy heart** may be caused by adhering too strictly, doggedly or obsessively to personal or social rules or codes of conduct (Hierophant), whether real or imagined (Moon).

12 THE HANGED MAN XII

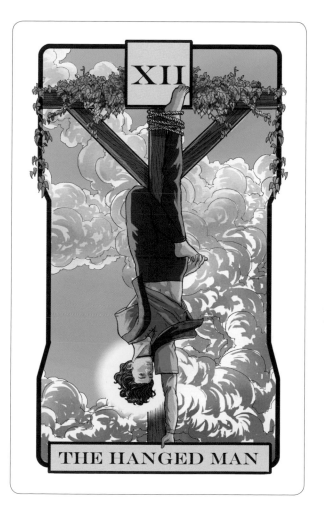

'To forgive is to set a prisoner free and
discover that the prisoner was you.'

LEWIS B. SMEDES

Personification – Psychology

The Hanged Man can represent a state of **psychological immobilization** after a significant ego assault (Tower, Death). When you have exhausted all attempts at negotiating depicted in the previous card (Justice) and have reached an irresolvable stalemate or impasse (2S), **total surrender** is your only remaining option: **relinquishing control** is the only way out of emotional pain and suffering.

Starting the process of **forgiving yourself and others** is key to this seemingly incarcerated archetype; 'for-giveness' means to give back or return any ego-assaulting energy, rather than allow it to continue to delineate your life experience. It's only by taking time out to **recognize and disown the original source of the emotional wound** that you can truly be released from it.

The great Indian independence activist Mahatma Gandhi, who himself spent lengthy periods of time immobilized in jail, once said, 'The weak can never forgive. Forgiveness [Judgement] is the attribute of the strong.' From this we can understand how this archetype, in their weakened position, **needs nothing other than time** – time to build the strength and resolve to truly forgive and set themselves free.

In the Hanged Man card, part of the elaborately structured ego scaffold still remains in place, though it is much reduced. The ego has not suffered a complete and total collapse. Instead it is left hanging by a thread, forced to utterly and completely relinquish its former dominant levels of cognitive control. Pulling out all the scaffolding at once would initiate a sudden structural collapse (Tower) and complete dissolution of the ego would result (Death), which, unless you are consciously and spiritually prepared for it, can constitute what the medical profession labels a nervous breakdown (Moon, Tower). It is only after this protracted period spent upon the Hanged Man's scaffold, angry, hurt and grieving, that **the old self is sacrificed** so any limiting or destructive aspects of the psyche are transmuted or transcended.

In **surrendering to what is** and remaining passive and inactive, you undertake a voluntary period of waiting, of allowing rather than actively trying to make your dreams and ambitions come to pass. The beautiful orchestrations of this archetype can be seen in how your external environment and events outside your control enforce a significant **pause to reconnect with your deeper desires.** Only when your thoughts are aligned with your greater potential will the timing be right for the next phase of your life to commence.

Depending on your perspective and psychological response, the inextricable experience of waiting and wanting can be easy and pleasant or uneasy and unpleasant. A waiting or wanting period can either feel like **a major setback or delay,** like you have been left 'hanging' or 'in suspense', or **a welcome rest and break from life's major or mundane concerns.**

Fighting or pushing for a desired outcome when external factors for its manifestation remain unaligned can cause unnecessary suffering. When this archetype appears in a reading, action or activating thoughts are futile. Nothing can be done to advance your cause, except **patiently and passively waiting, not wanting, for your life and its destined path to reconfigure and align** (Wheel of Fortune).

Sun Tzu wrote extensively on the art of the Hanged Man in *The Art of War*: 'He will win who knows when to fight and when not to fight . . . He who is prudent, and lies in wait for an enemy who is not, will be victorious . . . If you wait by the river long enough, the bodies of your enemies will float by.' In the modern sense, these 'bodies' can be viewed as the oppositional forces, both internal and externally mirrored in your surrounding environment, that are working against the manifestation of your greater potential.

In allowing an uneventful period of time to pass by, you are being provided with an opportunity to review your life (1S). **Waiting, withdrawing, stepping back or allowing things to settle themselves (4S)** is often a well-disguised blessing. **The longer the delay, the better, finer and more enjoyable the final gratification can be.**

Spirituality and Philosophy

Akin to an adult telling a child when it is the right time to cross the road, a higher, divinely inspired force holds the Hanged Man back. Only by **surrendering to a higher level of consciousness,** either the voice of the higher self or the wisdom of a trusted spiritual counsellor or mentor (High Priestess, Hermit), can we find true and authentic support.

By letting go and submitting or surrendering to a higher purpose or fate (Wheel of Fortune), the Hanged Man's voluntary or involuntary **pause to reconnect (Moon, Hermit)** brings ever-greater embodied en-lightenment (High Priestess, Sun); only when the body is hanged upside down do we start to really renegotiate the psychical weight we are carrying.

The Hanged Man on his cruciform-type scaffold evokes the image of Jesus being sacrificed on the cross and publicly shamed, yet the figure is turned the other way round seemingly remains there out of choice, suggesting a more private name-and-shame game is in play. Whether public or private, the more attention and energy are brought to the cause, the greater the opportunity for psychical refinement. To quote Confucius, 'The faults of a superior person are like the sun and moon. They have their faults and everyone sees them;

they change [Wheel of Fortune] and everyone looks up to them.' Thus the public or private exposure (Sun) of our mistakes or indiscretions (Fool) **subjects the arrogant, wayward aspect of the self to a greater blast of discrimination and, ultimately, refinement,** which fast-tracks our spiritual progress and evolution.

By voluntarily subjecting ourselves to some form of private or public exposure, we take a practical step towards subduing pride and arrogance (Strength) to cultivate deeper spiritual reverence, humility (Temperance) and eventually enlightenment (Magician, High Priestess, Sun).

Personal Life

The presence of this archetype in a relationship reading suggests **you need not rush into anything** with a new partner (1C, KnC) and that it might be more prudent to **slow things down** by delaying any official exclusivity agreement such as buying a property together (4W), accepting a marriage proposal (2C) or having children (Aces, Pages).

If the ball seems permanently stuck in someone else's court, it may be they are toying with you (2P) or **keeping you hanging as their 'undecided' option.** If this is the case, **completely disengaging from the object of your affection is better than waiting for them to re-engage with you.**

If you are already committed, your relationship could be going through **an inactive, uneventful, left-wanting or waiting period, or you might be voluntarily sacrificing a fundamental part of yourself** to keep yourself and another person tracking together. If one or both of you are having to make **major life compromises or sacrifices** to remain in your relationship, then this is best addressed sooner rather than later, lest any resentment build to a critical point, abruptly forcing the final dividing faultline (Death).

Professional Life

When this archetype appears in a work or career reading, it is likely that you will be voluntarily or involuntarily **surrendering, resigning or relinquishing control** to external sources or the powers over and above you. It could be that something out of your hands is holding up a project or work initiative, that **yours or another's hands are tied, or that nothing can be done to resolve an embargo.**

You may have devoted a significant amount of time or extreme amount of effort and energy (10W) towards higher learning (Hierophant, High Priestess) or fine-tuning or perfecting your craft (8P), or have put something out into the world and been **left in lengthy suspense awaiting a critical or public response (Judgement).**

If you have been passed over for a promotion, the Hanged Man philosophy is to just **patiently wait: when the time is right, all the external factors will align to provide a step up in your professional life (Aces).**

The Hanged Man-**style suspense** can be utilized brilliantly in the crafting and execution of dramatic tension (5W) in musical, creative, film or literary arts (Empress). Novelist Ruth Rendell explained how mastering **the art of maintaining a mystery** (High Priestess) via suspense was the key to her success: 'Suspense is my thing. I think I am able to make people want to keep turning pages. They want to know what happens. So I can do that.' This creation and maintaining of a suspenseful mystery (High Priestess) can be applied to any form of work that needs to **keep the public engaged, interested and wanting more over a protracted**

period of time. In the modern era, when gratification is becoming ever more instantaneous, holding an audience's attention, like holding a yoga pose, is a worthwhile challenge. But with the Hanged Man present, you will be able to **hold on to something or hold back and drip-feed** your audience, public, clientele, staff or colleagues as masterfully as the most suspenseful of fiction writers.

Property – Finances – Resources

In a reading regarding finances, the presence of the Hanged Man suggests there's **some form of voluntary or involuntary self-sacrifice to be made.** This is **not a time for actively pursuing your material goals,** but rather a time to passively hang back and leave financial opportunities, such as new projects (Aces), stocks, shares, property and investments, to grow, develop and mature over time.

If you are trying to sell a product, property, idea or service, **waiting patiently can bring a better or more worthy offer** (9P, 10P). Any financial or material situation, no matter how over-stretched your finances, can be resolved by **simply waiting it out.**

Some aspect of your financial life could be in **a seemingly precarious position (Fool).** You may, for example, be forced to wait a significant length of time before a bank loan is finally approved (Judgement, 6P), a property sold (4W, 6P) or a legal matter justly resolved (Justice).

This archetype also represents **the significant time it takes to make a big financial decision** (Judgement). How long the decision is pending and whether it is worth the wait depends on whether the surrounding or outcome cards are positively or negatively toned.

Health and Well-being

After the putting to rights of any major health imbalance (Justice), **an involuntarily extended period of abstinence or self-sacrifice** might be necessary to get your health back on track.

If you are going through a protracted period of **feeling helpless psycho-emotionally, physiologically strung out, suffering incurable hang-ups or physically asking too much of yourself**, it may be time **reorient your perspective, and, like the upturned Hanged Man, look at your situation from another angle** while taking a back-seat approach.

This is especially useful to remember if, for instance, you're awaiting the arrival of long-overdue medical test results, or for the birth of a baby after a seemingly long pregnancy. **Appreciating what you have as much as what you have not,** at any given moment, is the path to true wholeness and happiness.

13 DEATH XIII

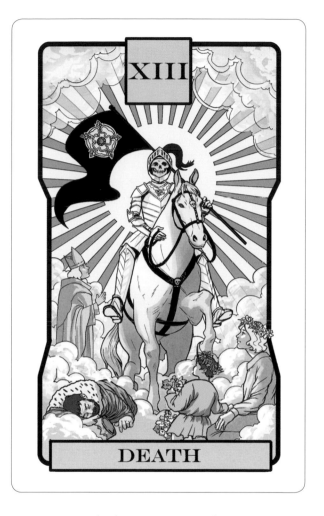

'Everybody wants to go to heaven,
but nobody wants to die.'
UNKNOWN

Personification – Psychology

On a mundane level, the Death archetype, as the conclusion of a major life cycle (Moon), symbolizes **a permanent and irrevocable change, ending, transition or transformation and the incursion of a great or significant loss.** Many years of fighting (5W) or resisting (7W, 9W) the tide of change have finally come to an end: **now is the time to give up the fight,** accept the end of this era and ready ourselves for the new one.

Of all things related to finality or endings, the **archetypal Death energy tends to frighten the rigid, anti-change aspect of the psyche** more than anything. Even when living in less than ideal circumstances, perpetuity is often preferable to the **destruction and upheaval** of this archetype. It is only with the benefit of hindsight that we can understand the higher purpose and design behind what initially appears to be **a merciless clearing and cleansing process.**

Though majorly unsettling, the Death archetype is a necessary stage in moving towards the sort of **major 'breakthrough' realizations (Judgement)** that can completely transform our life. For those who are able to push through their resistance to accepting Death as a crucial part of the grand cycle of change, there is the potential for a smoother transition to a brand new life.

Profound and lasting peace of mind (Temperance, Moon) can only be experienced when we learn to adopt an attitude of acceptance, appreciation and gratitude towards **natural cycles of ending and beginning.** By gracefully accepting (Strength, Temperance) that **all things must come to an end,** and even making preparations by clearing the way, we can harmoniously usher in a new chapter of life and all the new environments, people and characters that brings with it (Aces, Pages).

When the Death archetype appears, the most important battle to win is not with others, but with ourselves. Sun Tzu said in *The Art of War*, 'When your army has crossed the border, you should burn your boats and bridges, in order to make it clear to everybody that you have no hankering after home.' Though he meant this as a show of confidence in his army's ability to win, it was also a clever strategy in psychologically priming them for success. By **severing our attachments to the false safety and security nets of the past (Moon)**, we find a deeper wellspring of self-reliance and self-assurance (Hermit), of the type that can see us through anything. By fully **accepting what is gone,** and even helping to implement the transition, **we psychologically reset and reprogram ourselves for ongoing happiness, contentment and success.**

When the Death card appears, life may seem like a perpetual winter, and yet with just a subtle degree of change in approach, spring will appear, bringing new life with it. By allowing the fear of an ending to control our mood and temperament (Moon), our **negative thoughts and imaginings can make the experience worse** than it need actually be (9S). Fear-based decisions and actions taken (Moon, 8S, 9S, 9W) to try to avoid an inevitable ending only prolong (Hanged Man) and reinforce the suffering (10W). Any ending becomes more difficult as a consequence of active or aggressive (5W) resistance (7W, 9W).

Unless cards are present indicating the necessity of publicity (Sun, 8W), it may be more energy-efficient to keep the psychic death and rebirth cycle a wholly private process (High Priestess), lest attention precipitate external drama or conflict.

Spirituality and Philosophy

This card should be understood as the key aspect of the psyche's natural and cyclical (Moon) destructive-creative reconditioning process: death (10S), deconstruction (**Tower**) and rebirth or reconstruction (Star, Aces). Only by enduring our own **metamorphic death and disintegration (Tower)** can we progress to the next level in life, **purified, refined and en-lightened of the heavy lessons of life's previous cycle (Magician, High Priestess, Star, Sun)**. Like the primordial serpent of myth and legend, **our psyche sheds its skin in this continued process of self-renewal,** which allows it to be reborn afresh (Star, Aces). Death is but the final dramatic event of this stage-by-stage revelation process, as our consciousness is purified and realigned with its mother, the higher, nourishing light of the Divine (Star, Sun).

Personal Life

To fixed relationships, the Death card indicates a sudden, **forced** and often catastrophic **ending of a major relationship,** such as a divorce or the separation of close family and friends. When this archetype appears, a relationship has **irresolvable problems and the bond of love is damaged beyond the point of repair,** and any attempt to try and mend (8P) it, however sincere, is likely to be in vain (5C, 5S, 5W, 5P). At this stage, harbouring any falsely imagined (Moon, 7C) sense of security in a relationship, or even seeing a marriage or relationship counsellor to try and fix things (High Priestess), is just delaying **an inevitable ending.**

In some situations, divorce (Justice) may feel like **the ultimate release or final eradication of a non-nourishing, non-supportive, non-validating partnership.** We often allow the continuation of negatively impacting relationships for entirely the wrong and ultimately self-defeating (5S) reasons: fear of not finding anyone else (9S); habitual comfort (Moon); social expectations (Hierophant); to avoid social shame or the renunciation of our identity as a husband or wife (Sun). Whatever the reason, when this card appears for you, your acceptance of these self-defeating aspects (5S) are precisely what is holding you back from having a truly meaningful and satisfying relationship. The presence of this archetype indicates that the love, joy and comfort of your previous partnership are gone, making this **the ideal time to rise from the ashes of that relationship, full of potential like a brilliant newborn phoenix (Sun, 1W).**

If you are single, this card indicates **an emotionally difficult but necessary period of transformation.** It may be that via a lack of self-worth or self-esteem you repeatedly bring about **a dramatic end to relationships (Moon, 8S, 9S).** Having a **doomed-to-fail consciousness,** perhaps conditioned by the break-up or unhappy state of your parents' or caretakers' relationships, is another form of self-sabotage (8S). **Continually preparing for the worst, expecting things to end badly (9W) or falsely imagining yourself unworthy of love (Moon, 3S)** will mentally attract and manifest (Magician) the exact situations and people that will fulfil such negative prophecies. The physical world reflects back exactly what you imagine yourself worthy of or allow yourself to experience (Moon, 7C).

Professional Life

The presence of the Death archetype in a work or career reading indicates a major ending, like **leaving or being made redundant from a job,** perhaps one you have been in for a significant period of time. However, when a stagnating (8S) work situation ends, it enables an 'Onwards!' revolutionary movement (Wheel of Fortune).

In business, Death indicates that a company has either **merged with another and formed something new (Aces) or lost everything**. They may still remain in operation, but as a completely transformed version of what existed previously.

The presence of this card could also mean that your high hopes, dreams and expectations for yourself, others, a project or product have not been realized. Though your ideas, products or creations may have made it to market, it could be that changing times (2P) have rendered them too **quickly out-of-date, redundant or obsolete (Pages, 10S, 5P)**.

Many businesses and professions, in one way or another, profit from negatively impacting or emergency 'life and death' situations – lawyers, medical practitioners and military personnel, to name but a few. Thus when this archetype appears, it may also indicate that you are required to work in a service role, picking up the pieces of an emotionally or physically painful and distressing situation. However, the Death incurred may relate to animate objects that are suddenly rendered inanimate, like household boiler or vehicle breakdowns.

Property – Finances – Resources

The presence of the Death archetype in a finances reading usually indicates **insurmountable financial struggles and challenges or the incursion of a great or significant material loss.**

The stakes are as high as can be: **speculations, investments, stocks and shares are set to fail or do very badly** and the advice of this archetype is: 'Don't play the game if you can't afford to lose.' In total disregard for the materially acquisitive nature of human programming, this archetype works to **undermine all of** our previous material efforts. However, from a spiritual perspective, the major material or financial loss incurred via the Death archetype can be **an unparalleled liberator (Fool, World), forcing us out of chronically fear-driven (9S) material conformity (Hierophant) or habitual life repetition (Moon), stifling boredom (4C), suffocation and stagnation (8S).** Ironically, having nothing left to lose, or no financial constraints, gives us back the most precious and valuable thing of all: **complete and total freedom** (Fool).

The Death archetype can also indicate that a sad or unwanted situation could turn to your financial or material advantage, for example receiving **a life-changing inheritance or a big redundancy payout (10P)** when you were planning on leaving your job anyway. However, there is a warning against trying to engineer a fallout or disaster (Tower) that will be to your financial advantage (Devil), as this type of energetic input rarely goes unnoticed or is worth the eventual fallout (Justice, Wheel of Fortune).

Health and Well-being

The presence of this card in a health reading **indicates a sure need for healing people and environments.**

It can represent losing an inner battle to quit smoking, alcohol, drugs, abusive or destructive tendencies, or any situation inducing **chronic emotional distress, depression, psychological problems, phobias or suicidal feelings (Moon).**

A miscarriage, the voluntary termination of a pregnancy or the putting to sleep of a beloved pet (3S) may have left you feeling sad and bereft (5C). However, it is important to remember that this archetype rarely represents our own or others' physical death. It usually indicates the end of *a* story, rather than *your* story. What this card does always indicate, though, in one way or another, is **the absolute end of a battle, the peak moment of pain and suffering before life resets and takes a whole new shape.**

14 TEMPERANCE XIV

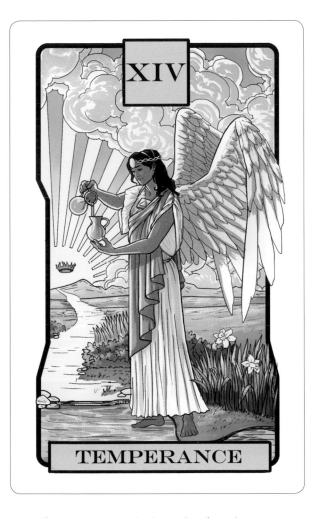

'If one oversteps the bounds of moderation,
the greatest pleasures cease to please.'

EPICTETUS

Personification – Psychology

The Temperance archetype's greatest long-term success is realized via their **ultra-tolerant, easy-going, open-minded, lenient, patient, accepting, controlled, ordered, adjusted, regulated, balanced, tactful, calm, restrained, diplomatic, equitable personality.** Nothing can rattle or shake this archetype. They **retain their composure and produce a measured response** to any drama or crisis, no matter how distressing the situation or how heightened the emotions of others (Death, Tower).

As a result of their **moderate words, feelings or actions, Temperance personifies elegance, charm and refinement,** even more so than the Empress archetype, which realizes these qualities only on a superficial level via privileged material and financial comfort. The Temperance archetype is **refined, balanced and harmonized to their very core, living in time and at one with all that is.**

Temperance comes from the Latin *temperantia*, meaning **'moderation', 'sobriety', 'discretion'** and **'self-control'**, and from *temperans*, the present participle of *temperare*, meaning 'to moderate' when applied to reactions and responses, behaviour, perspective or outlook.

When the eighteenth-century political activist and philosopher Thomas Paine said, 'A thing moderately good is not so good as it ought to be. Moderation in temper is always a virtue; but moderation in principle is always a vice,' he highlighted the importance of their card's positioning in a layout (as the crossing card read it as a vice). Due to its **moderate, regulating and restrained** appearance, ultra-ambitious individuals may not consider this card conducive to furthering their cause, whatever that cause may be. Looking at it through arch-rationalist eyes, such as those of seventeenth-century French author François de La

Rochefoucauld, who said, 'Moderation is the feebleness and sloth of the soul,' or nineteenth-century British prime minister Benjamin Disraeli, who said, 'Moderation has been called a virtue to limit the ambition of great men, and to console undistinguished people for their want of fortune and their lack of merit,' which in the crossing card position would be true. However, when placed otherwise, we can see how such ideas would appeal to the arrogant or overly robust ego and miss the finer point of this card altogether.

Far from being lacking in ambition, the **higher-minded ambition of this archetype is the cultivating of psychic integrity, which seeks to regulate our wayward, proud, arrogant, egotistical, degenerate impulses** and bring them into alignment with our greatest good, happiness and contentment.

The Temperance archetype understands how we measure personal success and what constitutes lasting satisfaction. Though material acquisitions or physical accomplishments can contribute to our happiness and sense of personal fulfilment, it is our ability to achieve **internal balance, agreement and constructive cooperation with ourselves and others that is the archetypical 'happy medium'** denoted in this card.

Spirituality and Philosophy

The presence of the Temperance archetype in a reading indicates **balancing your spiritually and materially driven psychic forces, thus enabling your will and decisions to be heart-centred, balanced, refined and therefore aligned with the higher, clearer, purer truth of the Divine.**

The phrase **'Know thyself'**, as we have seen (High Priestess), refers to self-awareness being the first step towards enlightenment. The by-product of this is a temperate attitude – a necessary prerequisite of entering a sacred space, such as the Temple of Apollo at Delphi. Thus it suggests that **the cultivation of a temperate nature is crucial to accessing the sacred space within; that it is only when we approach things in a balanced and refined manner** that we come closer to the energetic frequency of the Divine, the Great Creator: God.

Personal Life

Temperance is the antithesis of obsessive, fantasy or emotionally or socially ungrounded relationships. **Temperance takes their time to get the measure of any potential partners,** quietly putting them to the test to fathom if they are a good fit for them or not. Casual dating or seeing someone in moderation is also likely when this archetype makes an appearance.

Temperance indicates an **emotionally balanced and neutral relationship, where diplomatic harmony reigns through one or both parties rising above the fray.** Longer-term success is assured when we keep our emotions grounded by finding the appropriate response to any given situation. **Seeing things from the higher perspective of the Temperance archetype is the surest way to keep the peace.**

Professional Life

Temperance represents any work situation where **careful handling, coordinated cooperation, diplomacy, negotiating, deal-making or accommodating others' ideas and input** will pave the way for the greatest of successes in the long run. It represents colleagues **working together, despite any differences of opinion;** finding, positioning or reorienting yourself and others towards the middle ground; and **uniting any opposite forces in the workplace**. With this archetype, rigidly adopted positions or attitudes (Emperor) soften to produce **greater collaborative efforts via the harmonious integration, mixing, incorporation, combination, amalgamation or assimilation of others' ideas, projects and initiatives (3W), or skills and abilities (3P)**.

Temperance takes a piece by piece, one step at a time type approach: testing, assessing, checking, investigating, analysing, trying out, normalizing, delimiting, structuring, planning, measuring, standardizing, policing, ordering, synchronizing and making the out of range more accessible.

The measured and grounded approach of this archetype makes for great editors, accountants, mathematicians, doctors, scientists, lawyers, teachers or members of **any profession working in a measured way or 'by the book'**. It can indicate **finding common ground or the equitable conclusion** of any battle, disagreement or dispute (5W), legal (Justice) or otherwise.

Being risk averse, this archetype symbolizes taking **a centre-ground position** in all matters pertaining to the politics of work and business. But any implied mediocrity in the safe and sound appearance of this archetype is negated by the **awe-inspiring psychic integrity and mastery in the grounding and tempering of self-expression, desire, passion, enthusiasm and attachment** that are the basis for their success.

Ambition can wear many faces. The accumulative ambition of the Emperor, driven by intelligence, or the Empress, by creativity, can't compare or compete with the **balance and higher wisdom-driven ambition** of Temperance.

When entering a new line of work or studying a new subject, this archetype really takes the time to find out what is right for them before committing themselves to any long-term contract or endeavour. **They symbolize all low-risk and low-maintenance situations and people. They excel at minimalizing risk and** therefore represent all ventures that require only a minimal input in terms of time, energy and resources. They themselves make perfectly measured and calculated movements, never do anything to excess, and use only what they need and no more.

Though the rewards of their moderate endeavours may not be seen immediately, the overall success of their approach will be realized in the long run.

Property – Finances – Resources

The Temperance archetype indicates a sensible, balanced, precise, careful and considered approach to finances. They hate extravagance and excessive or wasteful spending. 'Try before you buy' is their modus operandi. This is the card of putting down deposits, holding fees or paying in instalments before committing to any full purchases. It could mean renting first before making a big home purchase in a new neighbourhood, taking a new car for an extra test drive, speaking to teachers and viewing a school or college in person before paying the first-year fees, or employing someone on a trial basis before offering them a more permanent contract.

This archetype always lives within their means; their financial incomings and outgoings are safely balanced and secure. They have a good head for business; by doing their sums and only taking precisely measured or calculated risks, usually on low-risk, low-yield ventures, they tend to win big in the long run (10P).

However, never once risking your personal or financial safety and security can lead to a life of wondering 'What if . . .?' What if you had taken that loan to start your own business or used an inheritance to buy a piece of land to build a rental property rather than paying off your existing mortgage?

Temperance isn't completely averse to the idea of speculating to accumulate, but if it appears as a crossing card, indicating what is holding you back, it suggests that **being too cautious with investment opportunities is moderating your means.**

Unless other cards suggest lesser (5P) or greater fortune (10P), in a like-for-like fashion this archetype's **conservative estimates and expenditures usually reflect their safe or mid-range earning potential (KnP, 7P); though they do receive adequate, equitable and fair payment for their goods or services.**

Often the acquiring ego creates much internal unrest in striving for a more glorified material existence. Yet the Temperance archetype's ethos when it comes to such material acquisitions is, in the words of the minimalist architect Mies van der Rohe, 'Less is more,' meaning that the path of unconditional adequacy, or being content with what you have, is the faster and more efficient route to lasting happiness. Ironically, it is often when we truly give up striving for our material goals that we attain the very thing that was always underlying them: **the enrichment of our own immaterial self-worth.**

Health and Well-being

To understand exactly how **this archetype enhances and retains their high-level psychical integrity** we need to look to their discerning quality, which, being **bent on equanimity of mind and purpose, jettisons destructive emotions,** rendering their mind an inhospitable environment for them to flourish in. As a reflection of their temperate interior landscape, **Temperance then enjoys an equally calm, collected, contented, harmonious and peaceful external environment, which in turn promotes good health and well-being.**

Moderation is the key to a healthy life: rest, play, sleep, relaxation, healthy eating and drinking, balanced with physical and mental exertion. So, if you are very fit, this card means not over-exerting yourself; if you are very unfit, it means getting out and exercising more often to rebalance your physiology.

Fifth-century theologian and philosopher Saint Augustine once said, 'Complete abstinence [Hermit] is easier than perfect moderation,' and when this archetype appears in the position of the crossing card, it indeed indicates exactly this: that moderation is an issue or in some way tempting fate. 'All things in moderation' is *an* ideal, but, for the addictive or obsessive personality, ultimate and complete **self-restraint, control, discipline and sobriety are *the* ideals Temperance works towards.**

15 THE DEVIL XV

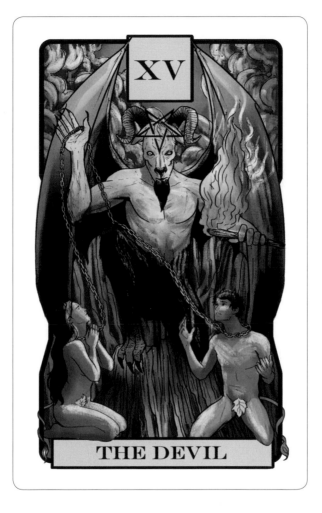

'If you tell a big enough lie and tell it frequently
enough, it will be believed.'
ADOLF HITLER

Personification – Psychology

The Devil archetype represents the **unpleasant consequences** we suffer by putting aside grace, virtue and good sense (Temperance, Strength) in the pursuit of **wild, base, ego-driven desires, entertainment and indulgences.** These can include: **immorality, wickedness, wrongdoing, iniquity, injustice, villainy, impurity, corruption, misconduct, sinfulness, stealing** (7S), **physically** (5W) or **emotionally** (5C) **wounding** (3S), **intimidation, manipulation, slyness, jealousy, envy, vanity, arrogance, greed, lust, perversion, debauchery, criminality, transgression, offence, vice, obsession, selfishness** (4P), **negativity, trickery** (Magician), **deceit, misrepresentation, misguidance, duplicity** (2S, 2P), **dishonesty, disrespect, degradation** (5S), **fear-based limitations** (8S) **and angry or violent conduct** (5W).

As a metaphor for our psychic processes, the Devil **corrupts, manipulates and compromises the integrity** of the other cards in a reading just like a virus or malware infects computer software. Surrounding cards will still operate as normal, as their basic qualities remain the same, but their energetic input will be utilized by the Devil archetype for **unhealthy and destructive purposes.**

To provide an idea of the corruptive nature of this archetype, using a political theme that could apply to many life situations, I have produced the following fully synthesized reading using a random selection of other cards:

Poorly informed individuals (Fool) announcing 'better ways' to run their country or national government often regurgitate (5S, 7S) attention-grabbing headlines from publications and newspapers (Sun) that rely on their sensationalist shock-value (Tower) and purist tone (Sun) **to manipulate the public,** promote false ideas and fulfil corrupt political or self-seeking agendas.

Political or not, the Devil represents those who, instead of using well-reasoned arguments, repeat attention-grabbing, headline-type slogans to **hypnotically promote their cause (Sun, 8W)**. Genocidal Nazi dictator Adolf Hitler (KW) openly admitted to the use of such brainwashing when he divulged, '**All propaganda [8W] has to be popular [Sun] and has to accommodate itself to the comprehension of the least intelligent of those whom it seeks to reach [Fool, Pages].**'

Writer Noam Chomsky alluded to the self-referential irony of the political spin doctor when he wrote, 'Remember, weapons of mass destruction don't mean missiles.'

The Devil can be seen in all false preachers (Hierophant) of **cultural, social or worldly purity (Sun)** who profess to be working towards the betterment of the world while failing to realize that they promote (8W) the very impurity they seek to snuff out.

Shock-value dramatics or theatrics designed to seize our attention (Sun) by diverting, deflecting and submerging our conscious awareness only further removes us from the natural state of equilibrium (Temperance) in which actual truth can be accurately and clearly perceived (High Priestess, Sun).

British prime minister Sir Winston Churchill, who successfully led Great Britain through the Second World War and helped to defeat Adolf Hitler (KW), once said, '**Can a nation remain healthy, can all nations draw together in a world whose brightest stars are film stars?**' Similarly, the Devil archetype gives **an indication of how, where and why our own mental health is compromised.**

The Devil's energy is seen most clearly in the divisive actions (5W) of showy, attention-seeking individuals (KW, QW) and an audience who values their dramatically or theatrically staged

arguments (Sun, KnW) over those that are clearly, cleverly and logically validated and articulated (KS, QS), kindly and compassionately motivated (KC, QC), and grounded in practical, material reality (KP, QP).

'Cosmic Comic' Swami Beyondananda perfectly summed up the Devil's psychology in his 2003 'State of the Universe' address, when he said, '**In the reptilian brain, problems aren't solved – they're attacked [5W].**'

In seeking to solve problems via their **vicious, dark,** murky, shadowy, ego-eclipsing actions, the **reptilian** Devil archetype contradicts themselves, adds complexity and confuses the issue. **A spin-doctored eclipse of the truth (Sun) is often used to promote the ego's self-validating narrative (Sun, Moon),** such as 'I am the hero who will save you.' Except only a false hero devises the very situation in which their victims then need saving.

When Indian scholar Swami Sri Yukteswar said, 'Some people try to be tall by cutting off the heads of others!' (10S), he perfectly captured the endemic prejudice of the undeveloped, immature and insecure personality. Unfortunately, the 'cutting off' of others' heads (10S) via racism, classism, chauvinism, sexism, anti-Semitism, etc., actually leads to those trying to make themselves feel taller and more empowered feeling smaller and disempowered.

Those who have been **socially or professionally bullied (5W), ostracized (Hermit, 5P) or who are suffering the effects of false accusations or character assassinations** should, above all else, attempt to cultivate a compassionate attitude (Temperance) towards such ego-led social executioners. Such people, when they select you as worthy of their destructive and jealous attentions, paradoxically **deepen their own social insecurities.** It is, I believe, the great paradox of the Devil archetype that behind all their outwardly diabolical activity lies **the subtlest, most convoluted, contradictory and convincing form of admiration and flattery.**

Spirituality and Philosophy

The tarot's **alchemical nature** in general, and the Devil card's in particular, are a great aid in **the deepest possible process of spiritual transmutation.** **Unrecognized shadow aspects** can only be dealt with when laid out in the open. Therefore, the very laying out of this card symbolizes the readiness of our psyche to be **filtered of any unintegrated shadow aspects by the refining light of conscious awareness.** Here we have the opportunity to become truly divinized (Star, Sun) by **purifying ourselves of all that is waywardly vile or foul.**

Receiving the Devil in a reading indicates that, at this time, **our progress is blocked by truth-opposing, unintegrated, degenerate or immoral aspects of the psyche.** These **unregenerate aspects,** like a dirty car windscreen that fails to show a true green light, only serve to **slow, delay and interrupt our journey through life.**

In a sense it is life, rather than the afterlife, that is **a purgatorial journey: a journey to expiate any ugly and bestial energies.** The Devil represents the pain and sorrow we must endure if we fail to reintegrate our shadow elements, which are indulged or entertained, to a lesser or greater degree, in all human beings.

Sun Tzu said in *The Art of War*, **'To know your enemy, you must become your enemy,'** and, **'The opportunity of defeating the enemy is provided by the enemy himself.'** Thus, by allowing the tarot to facilitate an honest dialogue with our shadow aspects, our psyche has the opportunity to reintegrate them and move closer to its goal of equilibrium, wholeness and completion (World).

Recognizing and labelling these aspects, proving we are aware (Sun) of their influence on our psyche, is the first step towards spiritual and, subsequently, earthly or material success.

The light of conscious awareness (Magician, High Priestess, Sun), when brought to **the dark and fearful psychic aspects** that oppose it, can vanquish even the fiercest of our inner demons. Like the fictional vampire, no dominant and controlling shadow aspect can survive the sunlit radiance of superhuman consciousness (Magician, High Priestess, Sun).

Personal Life

The Devil usually indicates a **dysfunctional, destructive and toxic relationship** that brings out the worst in all involved.

Unless you are a couple looking to spice things up via **bondage, domination, degradation or general all-round devilish sex**, then you may be tempted to do things that aren't for your greater good. Complying or colluding with someone's **negative, perverse, degrading, twisted, ruthless, devious, coercive actions or behaviour will be likely to result in a complete loss of your integrity and a sullying of your self-esteem** (Moon, 9S).

Those receiving the Devil in a relationship reading can be **suffering the ill-effects of domination, control, obsession, jealous rage, narcissism, inextricable co-dependency, lying, promiscuity** (Lovers), **cheating, two-timing infidelity, philandering** or a **duplicitous, illicit or unhealthy love affair** (Lovers, 2P, 7S).

The Devil indicates a situation in which someone is being **abused or exploited**, either sexually (Lovers), physically (5W), verbally (5S), emotionally or psychologically (5C).

If you lay out this card, it may be that you are in **thrall to a bad character**, someone who brings out the very worst in you. Their negative, fear-based thinking makes them act in a nasty fashion and harbour ill-will towards others.

In their shameless and insatiable pursuit of sexual indulgences, the Devil archetype also denotes a disempowering enslavement to the physical senses (Lovers). Thus their intentions are rarely based on love or respect. Extra vigilance is required around any charmer types (KnW, KnC), as the Devil denotes **those practised in the art of seduction.** As novelist Robert Louis Stevenson once cautioned, '**The Devil, depend upon it, can sometimes do a very gentlemanly thing [KnC, KnW].**'

If your independence or self-reliant nature (Hermit, KS, QS) is feeling challenged, you may even be dealing with the opposing **control-centric agenda of a narcissistic or obsessively co-dependent partner (Moon).**

Professional Life

'**Education without values, as useful as it is, seems rather to make man a more clever devil,**' said the novelist C. S. Lewis. The presence of the Devil archetype in a work or career reading usually indicates that morality or right behaviour is being sacrificed in the pursuit of worldly desires such as wealth, fame and respect. It could be that a corrupt or untrustworthy colleague has **a secret agenda to disempower you, or you them.**

This archetype **obsessively seeks absolute power, privilege and prestige (Sun), often via sneakily unearned leaps ahead (7S).** Their path to the top is marked by **studious obsessions, over-reaching or the over-amplification of ambition (10W)** to obtain a worshipped or celebrated career status (Sun), perhaps as some form of leader (Magician, Emperor), professor, teacher, preacher (Hierophant), or even intimate counsellor and adviser (KC, QC).

Like a sorry creature chasing its own tail, however, **the insatiable Devil archetype** finds the feeling of wholeness or completion, the closing of the circle (World), ever-elusive. Their inherent dissatisfaction and their devaluation (4C) of their accomplishments and achievements, no matter how great, **corrupt and compromise their own self-perception and subsequent sense of their own self-worth** through a perpetual feeling of lack or inadequacy.

If none of the above seems pertinent to your work situation, it may be that **devilish desire, perversity or that which exists only in the shadows of society and is culturally or socially prohibited** (Hierophant) is integral to your professional sense of self or the themes and identity (Sun) of your work.

Property – Finances – Resources

When C. S. Lewis said, '**The long, dull, monotonous [4C] years of middle-aged prosperity [Emperor, Empress, KP, QP, 10P] or middle-aged adversity [5P, 5C, 5S, 5W] are excellent campaigning weather for the devil,**' he pointed to the idea that the Devil archetype's **lust for and obsession with money and power** can keep us locked into a mundane, negative, detestable and ultimately joyless existence, whatever our material status. When we allow **our fixation on the material trappings** of life to own us, rather than the other way round, **seduced by the pleasures of the material world,** we find our life revolving in ever-tighter circles around the inanimate rather than the life-affirming.

The Devil is prone to **insecure or egocentric buying and spending.** They can arrogantly flash their cash to make themselves feel superior to others, though this only garners **ungratifying awe or respect** from those who are equally **immodest and insecure.**

By avoiding or shirking financial responsibilities and/or engaging in underhand dealings and illegal ways of making money or gaining resources, the Devil archetype tends to remain

forever insecure in their ability to access the visible upper ech-
elons of joy, happiness and abundance.

Health and Well-being

The Devil indicates choosing to stay in some form of **unhealthy
situation,** maybe a **self-destructive cycle or habit (Moon, 10S),**
perhaps out of **a stifling fear of change (Wheel of Fortune, 9S).**
If this card appears in a health reading, it may be that you have
relapsed into **dependent, addictive or destructive patterns and
behaviour,** abusing your mind and body by indulging your **physical senses** (Lovers) to temporarily escape a harsher reality
(Moon, 7C).

Having said this, the Devil's appearance in a reading does
offer a wonderfully liberating lifeline: the opportunity to rise
above **uncivilized impulses and instincts born of self-deceptive
ego-unconsciousness.** Only via truly honest self-enquiry (Magician, High Priestess, KS, QS, 1S) can you fine-tune (8P) and
eventually master (3P) those aspects of your character that will
ensure a brighter, happier and genuinely fulfilled future.

16 THE TOWER XVI

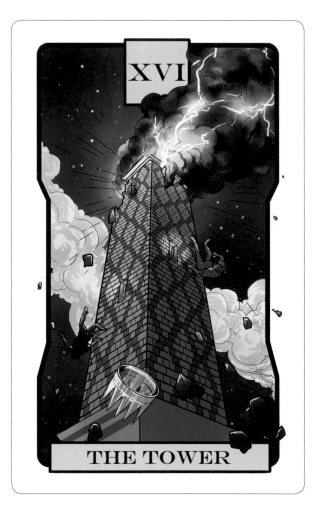

'Sceptre and crown must tumble down
And, in the dust, be equal made,
With the poor crooked scythe and spade.'

JAMES SHIRLEY

Personification – Psychology

When the Tower appears in a reading, longstanding things, assets, ideas, people and relationships are likely to break down and **disappear suddenly and unaccountably, making way for a brand new phase of life.** It's the proverbial cleaning of the slate, part of nature's great cycle of growth, change and transformation. How quickly, easily and painlessly we transition from one phase of life to the next depends on how we handle the Tower's **destructive upheaval, meltdown and complete collapse.**

The **destructive events** of the Tower are **designed to catch us off-guard,** so we are unprepared to defend, preserve, conserve and sustain whatever situation is stunting our personal development. Thus the **sudden, abrupt, unforeseen, unlooked-for, unintended, unanticipated, unplanned, surprising, startling, unlikely, improbable and accidental** strategy of this archetype is fundamental to its **devastating** success. The resulting **damage, destruction, disaster, catastrophe and calamity** of this card need not be feared: they are simply nature's way of removing us, forcibly if necessary, from a situation that is not serving our greatest potential.

When the Tower appears in a reading, there is likely to be something inauthentic about the way you are living, something antithetical to the higher ideals of truth, love, joy and happiness (Star, Sun). The Tower enacts **a sudden forceful blast of en-lightening truth** that forcibly tests, shakes and deconstructs some misaligned aspect of your life. The blast to the Tower's head indicates **the psychological shock and pain** when **unsustainable heights of pride, arrogance and self-conceit lead to self-destruction.**

As a force of nature, the Tower **redresses any great imbalances, enforcing humility and equilibrium (Temperance)** so we can action our higher, altruistic and self-less intentions with greater purpose and effectiveness. In accordance with nature's birth-death-rebirth, or, start-**destroy**-restart mandate (Wheel of Fortune), the Tower **enforces numerous transformations within** an individual lifetime. These are not physically destructive events, but rather **a virtual clearing and excavating of any numbing and obscuring ego-overlay (Moon, 10W, 10S)** to make way for the rebirth (Star, Aces) of a newly en-lightened psyche.

The higher design behind these repeated Tower cycles is **to disempower our fear-based attachments and insecurities by teaching us, via repetition, to be comfortable with uncertainty and vulnerability (Star).**

Buddhist nun Pema Chödrön highlighted the benefits of the deconstructive Tower aspect when she explained, in her teachings on *Cultivating Fearlessness and Compassion*, 'The **opposite of** *samsara* [the cycle of suffering] **is when all the walls fall down, when the cocoon completely disappears and we are totally open to whatever may happen [Star], with no withdrawing, no centralizing into ourselves . . . leaping, being thrown out of the nest, going through the initiation rites,** growing up [Hermit], stepping into something that's uncertain and unknown [Star].'

The Tower reflects our striving to return to that pure, comfortable, fearless, unconditioned point in our psychological history that Zen Buddhists, who follow the ideology of impermanence, call the 'beginner's mind' (Fool).

Spirituality and Philosophy

Although the Tower card may not initially appear to be a laughing matter, when American comedian Groucho Marx said, **'Blessed are the cracked, for they shall let the light in,'** he was, in essence, **prescribing the deconstructive joys of the Tower's vio-lent enlightenment process.**

The Tower **heralds the beginning of a deep spiritual initiation process, which can only commence once the integrity of the ego has been breached** by a shockingly powerful en-lightening force. Burning firelight is then seen through the Tower's two ocular windows, indicating **an enforced spiritual clarity of vision, both physiological and divinely metacognitive.**

When the Tower appears in a reading, you are on **the threshold of an initiatory experience (Star), a process of inner metamorphosis** from which you re-emerge as a brighter, higher and more divinized consciousness (Star).

The burning, 'purgatorial' hellfires raging inside the Tower, kindled by the preceding actions of the Devil archetype, lose their sting when we understand them as **a natural means of transformation** and surrender or submit to their **spiritual purification and purging.**

Alluding to the pain of resisting enlightenment by remaining in ignorance of yourself, Saint Catherine of Genoa once cautioned, '**The fire of hell is simply the light of God as experienced by those who reject it.**' Rather than resist and suffer, the Tower offers us the opportunity to purge that which seeks to tone down the glow of our conscious awareness.

If we are to be revitalized and initiated into a higher order of being (Star), the profane version of ourselves must suffer the psychic purification of the inferno that accompanies the Tower's archetypical fall from grace.

Over 600 years on, the echo of Saint Catherine's words in this book show her advice to be truly timeless.

Personal Life

The Tower in a relationship reading indicates **a big upheaval or sudden and unexpected change.** You are likely to be experiencing the **fallout from a bad or destructive situation,** perhaps bought about by an avoidance of the truth (2S), or are entrenched and immobilized by the fear of a big change (Wheel of Fortune, 8S).

What has been built up over time is suddenly crumbling. A longstanding relationship, such as a marriage, may be about to end (Death) or go through a major overhaul (8P); someone you previously counted on may no longer be there when you need them (Moon, 5C). This is **a chance to clear and reconstruct your personal life,** not just your relationship to others but also your relationship to yourself.

If you are single, **a new, true and authentic love (1C) may strike your life like a bolt out of the blue,** bringing your towering emotional defence structure (9W) tumbling down. **Only when our emotional defences are down** can any heart-to-heart connections be authentically revealed and established (2C).

Professional Life

The Tower in a work reading can be applied either in principle or practice. In practice it usually indicates **a loss of position, place, respect, power, authority, control, dignity: an involuntary dethroning, or the ideal time to voluntarily quit the arena.** When painter Salvador Dali said, **'Surrealism is destructive, but it destroys only what it considers to be shackles limiting our vision'** (Moon, 2S, 8S) and Pablo Picasso said, **'Every act of creation is first an act of destruction,'** they were referring to the

Tower's powerful **destructive-creative principle:** what the Chinese would similarly describe as **'finding opportunity in a crisis'** (Aces).

We even see **the Tower's destructive-creative potential** simplified in the commonplace saying attributed to eighteenth-century revolutionary leader Maximilien Robespierre: **'You can't make an omelette without breaking some eggs.'**

Another application of this card indicates work in **the emergency or crisis clearance services, demolition or deconstructive situations,** or even as some sort of cultural critic or an employer whose higher purpose behind **a destructive critique is to break something down so it can be rebuilt in a more effective or efficient way.**

However, a note of caution: this archetype can also indicate **the sudden and accidental loss of all your work, perhaps after a technological crash,** so be sure to back things up twice, or even thrice to be safe (4P).

Property – Finances – Resources

The Tower usually indicates **an intense financial struggle or a rapid and damaging transformation of your circumstances.** It could be that your **great expectations don't come to pass** or that uncontrollable forces and events have had a devastating impact on your bank balance. On a global scale (World) the Tower can indicate **a major economic crash or political or economic factors that adversely affect your own wealth and finances.**

By inflicting losses, the Tower seeks to address behavioural imbalances, such as the obsessive (Devil) pursuit of wealth and wanting to win no matter what the cost (Chariot, 6W).

However, applying the Tower's **destructive-creative principle** to property, the purposeful demolition or deconstruction of an old home can clear the space needed for a more efficient, effective or up-to-date rebuild.

Health and Well-being

The Tower indicates a **grievous or pressurized change, separation or severing of a deep emotional attachment.** It can indicate **a nervous breakdown or psycho-emotional collapse (Moon, 9S),** yet it is **only by breaking through (1S, 1W) and dissolving any old psycho-emotional structures, habits and routines** that we can begin the process of physically, mentally, emotionally and spiritually self-healing (Star).

Accidents and injuries such as broken bones, damaged muscle fibres or ligaments are often symptomatic of our internal struggles. Our conditioned reactions and responses to painful situations are to avoid and resist them. **But only by wholly facing the Tower's chaos and confusion can we avoid the helpless feeling of free falling and regain our lost sense of safety and security.**

The painful events of the Tower provide **an opportunity to reflect upon and understand the limitations of our own condition, then cultivate a balanced and unreactive attitude towards the inevitability of change.**

We can also help fulfil the Tower's mandate as an instigator of rebirth and profound identity **change (Star), by experiencing major surgery or deep therapeutic healing after a catastrophic breakdown.**

Physically, the Tower can indicate losing weight and the burn-off of bodily toxins, impurities and excess fat via an increased metabolism or energetic exercise (KW, QW, KnW). However, the purification process can also take place solely on a psycho-emotional level.

The ceremonial purification and ritual cleansing by fire of the forty-foot 'Man' effigy and Temple structures at the Burning Man Festival in the USA bears a striking resemblance to the scenes in the Tower. The Temple, akin to the Tower, is built solely for the purposes of **therapeutic release-healing** (Star). Event participants attach their expressions of grief, loss or triumph over adversity (Chariot, 6W), in note or photographic form, to the ephemeral wooden structure, which is then ritually burned at the culmination of the event.

Similarly illustrating the ideology of impermanence, the burning building depicted in the Tower archetype **urges us to free ourselves from pain and suffering by letting go of cravings and aversions to what is, from our present position, past or passing.**

17 THE STAR XVII

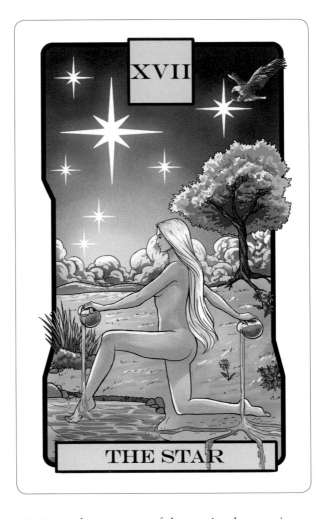

'It is not the strongest of the species that survives,
nor the most intelligent, but the one most
responsive to change.'

CHARLES DARWIN

Personification – Psychology

The Star-lit scenario often, but not always, is born of a Tower-type emotional trauma, which purposefully deconstructs and clears our life so our **more authentic core self is given a voice and, most importantly, the executive power of choice.**

Only by completely **opening, surrendering and relinquishing the aspects of ourselves that aren't honestly aligned with our highest hopes and potential** can we draw level with the stars. The English novelist John Galsworthy once said, '**Idealism increases in direct proportion to one's distance from the problem,**' so, when the problem is our old organizing structures or limited sense of self, either materially, emotionally, intellectually or spiritually, the quicker we let these go, the better (Tower, 10S). Only then can we more effectively **reconnect to our highest ideals and aspirations.**

The Star archetype **easily relinquishes and dissolves any fear barriers, parameters, restrictions or limitations (Moon, 9W, 8S)** that would otherwise block potential new or alternative life trajectories (Aces). Their **inherent low- or no-resistance attitude instantly re-identifies with any completely new changes of scene, identity, personality, status and profile to make things start happening for rather than against us (Magician, Aces).**

The archetypical Star energy **sees the re-connective synchronicities in the chaotic destructive-creative principle (Tower), and accepts and flows with whatever changes they bring as smoothly and easily as if we had purposefully pre-planned them. Rising above any personally limiting chaos, the Star's overview of the situation allows us to see the bigger picture or higher, geometrically measured design.**

The Star's **deep calm, contentment and healing** are made possible via this **higher-dimensional, geometrical reordering of our** otherwise chaotically non-compliant thought processes. They allow our lower mind to **reconnect with and replicate the thought patterns of the higher aspect of the mind,** so we can instantaneously understand the necessary steps to manifesting a purposeful and fulfilling life.

The scene on the card being **cloudless, coverless, naked as the day we were born** indicates the **newly emergent, penetrative, excavating, discovering and revealing** drives, impulses and concerns of this archetype. The Star encourages us to **relinquish any false conditioning (7S) and do what comes naturally, as per our individualized birth mandate,** by allowing the **deepest, most honest and authentic version of ourselves** to surface. There is no higher honour we can bestow upon ourselves than to openly live our greatest truth and share our surfaced soul with the world.

As the figure **humbly and penitently kneels** in awe of something far greater than themselves, we are also **encouraged to be thankful for the instructive hardships of the past that have brought us to this higher, clarified state of divine re-emergence.**

Spirituality and Philosophy

The Star archetype symbolizes **the enlightenment of the spiritual self; when, at the end of a dark time (Tower, Death, 10S), the dual aspects of the mind begin to converge towards the all-encompassing light.** One way or another, when this card appears, your life path has led you to the **dissolution of the ego and union or at-one-ment with the Divine.**

This archetype indicates **the re-routing of the conscious mind (Sun, Moon) away from the mundane or profane and towards more sacred or higher-minded concerns.** Thus, by disengaging from mundane earthly concerns (Strength), we can experience the **higher-dimensional unconditional** love, joy **and soul-surfacing of an en-lightened being.**

The Star card is characterized only by those in **the initial naked stages of self-realization,** when the newly surfaced soul is **laid bare for all to see.** The destruction of the concealing walls of the Tower has **left the false shadow aspect with nowhere to hide, nowhere to thrive. Opened to scrutiny, the spirit can be purged of all shadow forces, and all the wounds we have accu-**mulated can now begin to heal.

As an initiation begins by removing all personal clothing, jewellery and accessories, **the spirit is left symbolically naked, owning nothing but its thoughts, which can weigh heaviest of all when we are possessed by our own possessions.** In our stripped-back state, **we are invited to contemplate our values and to recognize, own and transcend the vanities and profanities of our existence.**

So **we begin to cast off the heavy, mundane concerns of the world and realign ourselves with the subtle, perfectly ordered evolutionary geometry of the unpossessed spirit.**

Personal Life

In a love reading, the Star refers to **new feelings emerging (1C).** Suddenly you can **clearly envisage what you want and start to make it happen (Magician).** The Star indicates **a true, authentic and trusting love relationship** or the epiphany that makes you **go the extra distance** to find this.

You may feel **inspired to come out and show the world or your partner who you truly are.** Having the courage **to show up in your entirety or be completely yourself,** minus the front or any guarded behaviour, reaps the greatest emotional rewards (1C, 2C, 9C, 10C). As a result, you may attract **someone who** makes you feel more yourself, as well as strong, secure and fearless (Strength). This is likely to be a natural partnership, where you feel secure in your vulnerability with the other person. Establishing and retaining absolute trust with a partner is archetypical Star-lit behaviour.

Star partners inspire you to be the best version or vision of yourself. You feel a deep, inexplicable spiritual connectivity to them. This is true, pure love minus the possessive craving and attachment.

Holding the highest vision of what you want in a partnership and not compromising or settling for anything less are crucial to your success. The 'one' will be likely to be beyond what you imagined them to be, someone who broadens your life trajectory. They may move you beyond the tick-box of the type you are usually attracted to; how and why you love them, like the universe, are likely to be ineffably felt rather than logically answered, indicating the heart-centred authenticity of your choice.

Professional Life

The Star points to synchronistic happenings and the cosmic timing of events bringing you what you most need or require. This is the right moment for something new to emerge (Aces), such as a project, product, service or the undertaking of a new work opportunity to rebuild, renovate or reinstate an outdated and dismantled structure or system (Tower).

The key to understanding this card is to think of its universal qualities, i.e. vast, mysterious, unknown and inexplicable, meaning the work you are starting now is bigger than you are, or part of a larger, divinely ordered and ordained system.

The Star inspires all highly creative risk-taking and breakthrough works of art, literature, invention and industry. Its inspired ideas are unique, original, innovative, inventive, experimental, novel, imaginative, creative, new, unusual and unprecedented; the stuff of the future; the grounding in material reality of speculative or science fiction.

Being ahead of its time, the future ramifications of the Star are shrouded in mystery. The divine inspiration of theoretical physicist Albert Einstein can be seen in his ever-open and enquiring mind, which found little comfort, stability or security in the 'known' universe. In his own words: 'The most beautiful thing we can experience is the mysterious. It is the source of all true art and all science. He to whom this emotion is a stranger, who can no longer pause to wonder and stand rapt in awe, is as good as dead: his eyes are closed.' Thus the Star refers to the classical *Sciencia*, the understanding of the infinite and immeasurable network of connections underlying all aspects of reality, rather than the modern Science of measured laboratory experimentation.

Echoing the motivational words of British prime minister Benjamin Disraeli, '**Nurture great thoughts, for you will never go higher than your thoughts,**' the Star, as **a great leap-enabling energy, allows us to reach heights never attained before.** If negotiating a salary, service fees or a pay rise, ask for more than you think possible, as the **results are likely to go way beyond your expectations (9P, 10P). Don't allow practical reality to limits your ideas** – go beyond what is usually possible. Through divine synchronicity and timing, the finances or resources you need are likely to appear, often from **an unseen or usually distant source (6P).**

Health and Well-being

In a health reading, the Star is a reference to being **healed, mended, regenerated, rejuvenated, reconstituted, regrown and reborn** after the previously destructive events of the Tower card.

The Star enables **positive changes in health or fitness routines, staying extra hydrated, flushing out toxins or releasing blocked energy in the body, or simply spending time in calm, soothing, tranquil, peaceful or meditative environments.** It indicates a **natural relinquishing of control and surrendering to the unknown;** what Pema Chödrön describes as being '**totally open to whatever may happen, with no withdrawing, no centralizing into ourselves** ... **stepping into something that's uncertain and unknown**'.

Cultivating the Star-bright attitude of working with rather than against the flow of life will replace any resistance or panic with a deeper-drawn sense of calm, contentment and harmony.

18 THE MOON XVIII

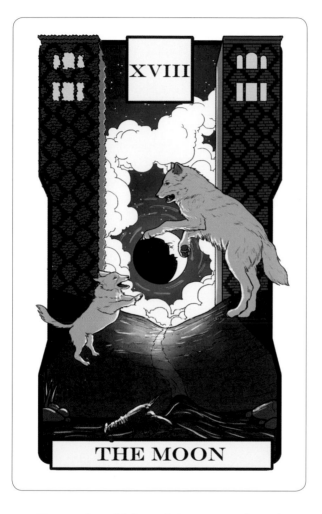

THE MOON

'In any city with lots of skyscrapers, lots of
skyline, the moon seems bigger than it is.
It's called the moon illusion.'

NEIL DE GRASSE TYSON

Personification – Psychology

The Moon projects and reflects our sense of self (Sun), as engendered by our psycho-emotional conditioning. Or, as René Descartes put it, 'I think [Moon], therefore I am [Sun].'

As a card of absorption and reflection, the Moon lends agency to the other cards in a reading, amplifying and empowering **self-absorption** (Sun, 4C); **acceptance** (Temperance); **accommodation** (Empress); **admiration, adoration, appreciation** (Sun, Emperor, Empress, Hierophant); **amusement** (3C, 4W); **anxiety** (8S, 9S); **awe** (Star, Sun); **awkwardness** (Hanged Man); **boredom** (4C); **calmness** (Temperance, Star); **confusion** (5W, 7C); **craving** (Devil); **empathy** (High Priestess, KC, QC); **entrancement** (Magician, Devil); **envy** (Devil); **excitement** (Sun, 3C, 4W); **fascination** (Devil, Sun); **equanimity** (Temperance, Strength); **fear** (Death, Tower, 3S, 8S, 9S); **horror** (Death, Tower); **joy** (Sun, 4W, 1C, 3C, 10C); **nostalgia** (6C); **passion** (Lovers, KnC, KnW); **reflection** (Hermit); **romance** (Lovers, 1C, 2C, 10C, KnC); **sadness** (3S, 9S, 10S, 5C, Tower, Death); **satisfaction** (9C, 10C, 9P, 10P); **sexual desire** (Magician, Lovers, Devil, 1W); **sentiment, sympathy** (Empress, KC, QC); and **triumph** (Chariot, 6W, 9C).

The Moon **represents the veils of interior projection, illusion and delusion, all our private, personal and subjective representations of reality**; what French author Anaïs Nin meant by saying, 'We don't see things as they are, we see them as we are.'

So the Moon's presence in a reading signals that **your expectations of yourself, another person or situation are being mirrored back at you.**

The Moon also points to all **unnecessary dramas in our lives** caused by our personal or psychological safety and security issues: overactive fear (9S), doubt, hesitation, confusion, uncertainty, misunderstanding, misrepresentation, mistrust, mis-communications and inconstancy, paradoxically occurring as habitual, repetitive or cyclic movements.

American astrophysicist Neil de Grasse Tyson spoke of the Moon's **potential for perceptive confusion**: 'Kids don't care about full moons ... They only get scared of magic or were-wolves [as a result of] ... stupid adult stories [7S].'

Under dubious, misguided, misleading, unfounded or imagined influences (Devil, Pages, Fool), the projecting, Moon-moved individual can quickly and easily jump to **a wrong conclusion.**

Fear-based reactions to the unfamiliar or unknown are the Moon's signature form of **illusory influence,** as in the ancient Greek philosopher Heraclitus' comment, **'Dogs, also, bark at what they do not know,'** which is illustrated here on the Moon card.

Taken to its extreme, **the Moon can separate and isolate us (Hermit, 8S)** from new, unfamiliar or foreign experiences – what we fearfully imagine to be insecure or unsafe people, places or positions. To live a truly secure and happy life, we must strive to become comfortable with the unknown.

The presence of the Moon in a reading signals that **any usual forms of physical, psychological or emotional support are influ-encing our life in an unfamiliar, non-protective or security-testing way.** This can be **a mother figure (Empress), a father figure (Emperor), offspring (Pages), family members, care providers, counsellors (High Priestess, KC, QC); nurturing benefactors; shelters, money lenders, funding sources (6P, KP, QP); informers, instructors, mentors, teachers, schools, schoolteachers, (High Priestess, Hierophant, KS, QS); institutional bodies, agencies of the establishment or governing bodies (Emperor, Hierophant); the habitual customs of a tribe or nation; parochialism, region-alism, patriotism, nationalism (4P); memories, the past, roots,** familiar faces or places: childhood friends and countrymen (6C); religious or institutional meeting-places, schools of thought, social conventions, folk and cultural norms or traditions; religion, (Hierophant, High Priestess); groups, societies, clubs (3C); eating and drinking customs (Empress); boats, vehicles (6S); the house, buildings (6C), walled structures or compounds that are secured, protected or defended; shells or personal boundaries (2W, 9W); safes, lock-ups, safety-deposit boxes (4P); physical protectors: the army, the police, security guards (Knights, Chariot, 9W); the law (Justice); customs officers and border police (Judgement, 9W).

What was once a familiar source of comfort and security has now become a source of worry and anxiety, or vice versa, depending on the positive or negative tone of the surrounding cards. Yet the Moon **instils fear, worry, anxiety and confusion** via its cyclical repetition of difficult or challenging events, to teach us how to **transcend them (Star, World): by cultivating our sense of familiarity with the unfamiliar (High Priestess, Sun).**

Spirituality and Philosophy

Though private and operating by night, **the Moon's mandate is to reveal and highlight all otherwise hidden, occulted, obscured or unconscious matters and truths (High Priestess).**

Being a night-lighting luminary, the Moon signals **our innate ability to see beyond the limitations of the material world (High Priestess) by cultivating our sensitivity and receptivity to gut-instinct, inner knowing, intuition, extra-sensory or psychic awareness, out-of-body experiences, and lucid or symbolic dream alchemy experiences.**

The Moon **enables our unconscious to leap over our slower cognitive reasoning. It produces intuitive answers to questions in**

176

a 'download' that appears as anomalous, 'out-of-nowhere' flash thoughts. The cognitive mind may try (and fail) to explain, unpick and undermine them. **When we quietly observe our mind's inner dialogue, we can clearly discern cynical, doubtful, logically and rationally calculated afterthoughts from the divinely assured clarity of intuitive forethought.** In shining a spotlight on the inadequate response times and dubious clarity of our cognitive mind, **we can actively disempower this slower, defunct aspect of our thinking and reinstate the clarified mind's speedy intuitive processor.**

Personal Life

The Moon in a relationship reading signifies the **comfort or discomfort we receive from certain partners or our familiar and habitual relationship patterns.**

The Moon also indicates a need to examine the complexities of our love life, **to straighten out any unhealthy attachments, clinging, addictions, obsessions (Devil), compulsions or aversions. By contemplating the hidden emotional forces in a relationship, which nevertheless exert power and influence over us, much like the Moon moves the tides, we can choose to ride our emotional waves rather than be dragged down or further out of synch by them (High Priestess).**

We can only cultivate sound love for ourselves and others when we rise above our fear of loss and rejection-based co-dependencies. In Shakespeare's tragic love story *Romeo and Juliet*, **Juliet Capulet stresses the dangers of her lover's dependent pledge of lunar love: 'O, swear not by the moon, th' inconstant moon, that monthly changes in her circle orb, lest that thy love prove likewise variable.'**

Yet, despite its **cyclical, unsettled, push-pull or tidal influence** on a relationship, coming and going, ebbing and flowing (2P), the paradoxical Moon, in its monthly regularity, can also symbolize **habitual continuity (2C): love's great dream grounded in mundane reality.**

Fortunately, the Moon's presence in a reading can help **turn any confusion to disillusion (4C). Once we realize a person or situation is not as we imagined it to be,** our imagination can work for rather than against us (Magician) and help us envisage a better future. As Anaïs Nin said, **'There are many ways to be free. One of them is to transcend reality by imagination.'** Then we can avoid the archetypal Shakespearean tragedy (Tower, Death, 5C).

Professional Life

In practice, the Moon can signify **work being erratically coming and going, ebbing and flowing (2P), devoid of any structure or routine, or a nocturnal or night-shift type arrangement.**

In principle, the Moon indicates **the degree to which we receive, absorb and reflect others' collective and projected expectations of us (7C),** which we can of course choose to refuse (7W), like actress Penelope Cruz, who said, 'I was eleven when I first said I wanted to become an actress, and everyone looked at me as if I had said I wanted to go to the moon.'

Due to its **reflective, receptive and familiar close-to-home nature, the Moon can indicate representational or performing roles,** such as actor (Sun, Fool, KW, QW), diplomat, ambassador (Temperance, World), figurehead or leader (Sun, Empress, Emperor, KW, QW): those we see regularly, whether we know them personally or imagine we do through the falsely engendered intimacy of our various forms of home cinema or media viewing platforms (7C).

It also signifies what is **hidden, unobvious or not in plain sight**, hence the thought behind any creative act, for what cannot be seen must be imagined.

The archetypical style of the Moon is **impossible, nonsensical, illogical, contradictory, paradoxical, puzzling, oxymoronic, enigmatic, constant and habitual vs inconstant and ever-changing,** which, when used for creative purposes (Empress), can prove highly entertaining; as the author Lewis Carroll's Red Queen said to Alice, in *Through the Looking-Glass*, 'Sometimes I've believed as many as six impossible things before breakfast.'

Property – Finances – Resources

The Moon's money methodology is simple: what will happen is wholly dependent on what you can imagine. But when making financial decisions, the Moon suggests that you need to **combine intuition and gut instinct with the analysing of facts and crunching of figures.**

On a practical level, the Moon also indicates whether your basic needs, such as food, water, warmth and clothing, are being met, and can highlight **shelter issues: the home, real estate, property ownership (4W) and home-building (8P).**

When this card is present, your **earning and spending may become erratic or compulsive, with money going out as easily as it comes in.** The temporary gratification of retail therapy may be playing havoc with your finances (5P), and when the Moon is surrounded by cards of lack or inadequacy (Hermit, 5P), you will find that **people or sources you thought could be relied upon for financial support are no longer able or willing to assist you.**

A key step towards the blissful state of spiritual liberation or en-lightenment (High Priestess, Sun, 1C), is in **the rejection of** materialism, or at least a cyclical clear-out of accumulated psycho-material junk. The finding of ultimate happiness by re-identifying with the divine immaterial aspect of life is echoed in the timelessness of Matsuo Basho's seventeenth-century poetry: 'The moon is brighter since the barn burned', meaning the purification and eradication of our psycho-emotional store-house.

Health and Well-being

The Moon in general indicates the mysterious ebb and flow cycles in life and health. As science fiction author Jules Verne noted, 'Numerous observations made upon fevers, somnambulisms, and other human maladies seem to prove that the moon does exercise some mysterious influence upon man.'

The ancient Vedic wisdom tradition of India *inextricably* links the Moon's movements with the ebb and flow of human emotion and the physical body's waterways or pumping systems: blood, circulation, the menstrual cycle, the glandular system, the urinary tract, etc.

On the other side of a far less connected nineteenth-century world, Irish dramatist Lady Gregory also intuited that, 'The time the moon is going back, the blood that is in a person does be weakening, but when the moon is strong, the blood that moves strong in the same way. And it to be at the full, it drags the wits along with it, the same as it drags the tide.'

Thus the Moon indicates the potential for mental burnout or emotional exhaustion (9S) caused by overwrought or 'knife-edge' emotions ruling over an otherwise stabilized mind. Moon-induced paranoia stemming from a restless or overactive mind and imagination can, if left unchecked, lead to involuntary social alienation (5P) and sleeplessness (9S), though under the influence of restful cards (Hermit, Temperance, Star, 4S), the Moon indicates the need for a period of **meditation, contemplation, introspection, reflection, respite and sleep.**

The Moon represents all mental or emotional health imbalances: hyper-awareness, alertness and perceptivity; emotion-driven overthinking, analysing, complicating and sensitivity (5W, 10W); depression, bi-polar disorder; hallucinations, paranoia, phobias, chronic fear and anxiety, insecurity, panic attacks; nightmarish dreams or **unhelpful fictional imaginings and narratives: the negative stories we tell ourselves (9S).**

In the cards surrounding the Moon we see **the consequences of its fixed or habitual emotional patterns:** obsessive-compulsive behaviour (Devil), psychological fear-based avoidance (8S), ego-projections (Devil, Sun, 7C) and compulsive eating disorders (Devil).

Whatever way our psychological or emotional security is feeling threatened or compromised, **seeking out professional support and advice (High Priestess, KC, QC) can help alleviate the fear-based symptoms of this emotionally minded archetype.**

19 THE SUN XIX

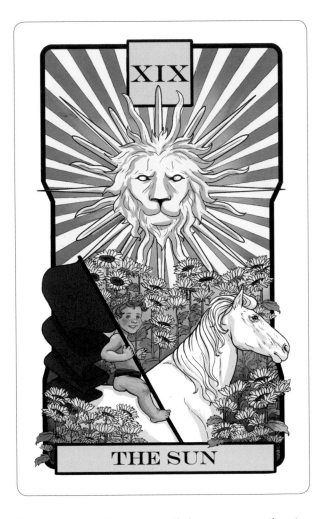

'The sun alone illuminates all this universe. Likewise,
the living soul, within the body, illuminates the
entire body by consciousness.'

THE BHAGAVAD GITA

Personification – Psychology

When the Sun archetype is present, whatever we were seeking has been found; we no longer simply believe we are on the right path, we know it. We have surrendered ourselves in full and can now experience the wisdom, love, joy and humanity beyond the walls of our own resistance (Moon).

The Sun represents what's highly visible, obvious and un-avoidable, and all things at the centre or concerning centrality, such as a powerful male or female public role model; personality; the public persona (KW, QW), the body's heart centre; births and beginnings (Aces); children (Pages), romance (Lovers), love (2C); public or iconic buildings and places, people, products, objects; the city; capital cities; bright lights, central or tourist attractions (4W); advertisements and headline news (8W); literal and figurative sources of power, government, politics; main events and attractions, sporting events (Chariot, 5W, 6W, 9C); special occasions, birthdays, parties, celebrations; the celebrated, celebrity, fame; theatre; royalty, ceremony; entertainment, amusements, performance art; applause, literature, music, dance, games, gambling (4W, 3C); creativity; teachers, professors, gurus (Hierophant); flamboyant, stand-out clothing, decoration, adornments; all things brilliant, radiant, hot, red, gold, shining and sparkling.

The Sun also symbolizes the beam of our conscious mind, as it radiates direct, brilliant, bright enthusiasm, motivation, hope, innocence, purity, virtuosity, confidence, courage, boldness, will-power, self-determination, drive, ambition, authorship, authority, autocracy, autonomy, individuality, independence, non-conformity and uniqueness.

When Indian sage Ramana Maharshi said, 'The bliss of the Self is always with you and you will find it for yourself if you seek it earnestly,' he was referring to the illuminating Sun principle bringing out our most authentic individualized expression.

The Sun is the energy behind those who exhibit self-knowledge and self-assurance; the vigour and flamboyance of royal confidence and radiant certainty, the certainty of a personality (KW, QW, KnW, PW) that makes no allowance for shyness, confusion, doubt, uncertainty, fear or ambiguity (Moon, KC, QC). Thus it does not mix or work well with those of lesser conviction or personality, and its self-confident, fun, exciting, showy or theatrically staged arguments (KW, QW, KnW) often outshine or eclipse those which are more cleverly and logically articulated (KS, QS, KnS), sensitive, caring and compassionate (KC, QC, KnC) or grounded in practical reality (KP, QP, KnP).

The Sun combines the pure, unadulterated, playful innocence of a child's mentality with the wisdom of the seer or sage who is living moment to moment with little or no care for the past or future, re-experiencing the childlike joy of being completely here, present and self-lessly enlightened (Fool, Pages). Yet, dualistically, the Sun can also show the way someone promotes themselves or their own self-interests (4P) in a way that is akin to the self-serving instincts of a toddler's 'Look at me' or 'I want . . .' need for validation.

The shining spirit energy of the Sun guards and protects the psyche by irradiating our unintegrated shadow aspects (Devil), burning off the impurities that fuel our wayward, profane or degenerate impulses.

The Sun seeks to highlight, put on display and make public all the other cards it appears with in a reading. Whether they are negative and ugly or positive and pleasing doesn't matter; the illuminating Sun principle alone doesn't discriminate. However, when paired with discerning and discriminatory influences (Magician, High Priestess, KS, QS, 1S), the Sun is capable of the greatest personal intelligence, wisdom and creative genius.

Spirituality and Philosophy

Free of any ego dross and impurities (Devil), the Sun is **the voice of the soul, higher self or conscience, enlightening the lower self with subtle knowledge and spiritual aspiration.** Its light, radiance, wisdom, perfection, truth and love are the celestial image of the divine consciousness in humanity.

Spiritual author and healer Edgar Cayce once said, 'The **strongest force used in the destiny of man [Wheel of Fortune] is the Sun.'**

The Sun symbolizes the **clarification, illumination and elucidation of ignorance or misunderstanding,** and yet too much Sun light (KW, QW) can blind us to subtle, spiritual or hidden realities: the area outside the arena or perspective platforms of life, or the mind. When our conscious awareness is directed only towards what is most central, visible and obvious, we effectively become Sun-blind to the spiritual dimensions of life. This is the unfortunate effect of the Sun or the Wands courtiers in the position of a crossing card.

The spiritual utility of this archetype is therefore wholly dependent on the presence of cards that convey a deeper sensitivity to or awareness of the hidden, subtle and multi-dimensional nature of reality (Magician, High Priestess, KC, QC). We need a balance of rational Sun and intuitive Moon energies if we are to manifest a balanced and fruitful life, a life which, as nature intended, grows only at night.

Personal Life

The Sun symbolizes a time of joy, happiness, enjoyment, love, light, faithfulness, contentment and freedom from restraints in a personal relationship (10C).

It can indicate a love relationship (2C, Lovers) or new emotional experience (1C) that is self-confirming, self-validating and highly pleasurable. This is likely to be a natural relationship in which you can be exactly who you are: your true, authentic self. The Sun archetype engenders highly expressive, dramatic or public displays and declarations of emotion or feelings (KC, QC), showing that you and a partner hold each other in the highest possible regard.

However, the Sun can indicate favouritism or being awe-struck by a partner. Be cautious of putting others on a pedestal; when you are blinded by their light, their faults can become imperceptible (2S).

The Sun can also symbolize an attention-commanding dynamic in a relationship (KW, QW), where one or both partners feel insecure unless they are continually celebrated, adored or in some way recognized for their splendour or magnificence. Though these partners can be a lot of fun, as is the nature of the theatrical, showy, dramatic or celebrated personality (KW, QW), they can also be selfish and self-centred. Thus the Sun-energized relationship often suffers and breaks down due to a lack of equality and diplomacy.

In its best and purest expression, the Sun indicates a partner who is generous, both financially and/or in investing a great deal of time and energy into the relationship (2C). If this is the case, it's likely you will be enjoying some fun times together, like parties or summer holidays.

If you are single and looking for love, the Sun signifies finding what you seek at a big, celebratory or high-visibility event (3C, 4W). Such are the high-visibility roles of the Sun that it can signify the bride or bridegroom on their wedding day, with all eyes upon them.

Professional Life

The key to understanding the Sun is that **nothing can hide from its light**; as such, the impulse of this card can draw you into **out-of-doors work or a work space with more exposure to sunlight**. However, the more likely interpretation is **self-promotion** or the public exhibition or exposure of your work efforts (World, 8W), whether intentional or not.

The Sun in a work reading often indicates the establishing of a dramatic, entertaining, **sunflower-like, head-turning** product, project, image or personality. Whether it is a commercial product's rise to fame (KP, QP, 3P, 10P), a literary or intellectual project's (KS, QS) marketing campaign (8W), a newsworthy politician's speech (KW, QW), or a sporting, music, art, film or theatre event, the Sun indicates a great and public accomplishment that is viewed as **the paragon of radiance and popularity (Magician, Emperor, Empress), the zenith of worldly recognition and success (World, 3P).**

Sun-influenced work roles include (but aren't limited to): the **publicly brilliant, famous, celebrated, halo-enshrined, crowd-pulling** type energy or **personality**; those with **celebrity-level vitality and charisma; high-visibility** careers such as those in the **performing arts** (KC, QC); **politics and public speaking** (KS, QS); **games** and **sporting events** (5W, 9C); **flamboyant creativity** or a **shining attractiveness** of performance, ideas or style that **magnetizes** the **interest** and **attention** of **the masses** (Empress, 3P); or those who take the **centre-stage role of guru,** mentor, preacher, professor (Hierophant); and the subjects of philosophy, politics and performance.

The Sun represents highly visible, independently acting **leadership roles (Emperor, Empress, KW, QW); highly charismatic** and **public** creative-writing projects (Empress); the **great minds** of history, such as the **Enlightenment philosophers (KS, QS); pure-hearted or corrupt (Devil) politicians; and generally anyone established and widely or publicly recognized.**

Rationality is strong with this archetype, but so are **purely self-interested objectives;** this may be fine in commercial matters, but not in situations relying on equality or diplomacy.

When the Sun appears in a reading, **this is the time to play with your biggest and most self-expressive creation or idea (Star, Empress, 3P).** It is the time to invent, experiment, grow, flourish and have fun doing it.

Property – Finances – Resources

The Sun is usually a card signalling prosperity and abundance. As the nourishing source of all growth in nature, **the Sun cultivates both the vision of what you desire and the belief in yourself that allows it to happen.**

The key here is publicity. It could be that a project, investment or speculation (Strength) draws **a lot of public interest and attention, so the generous revenue or financial rewards you receive from it exceed your expectations (10P).** This could be the launch or stock listing of a company you have a significant stake in (Aces).

The Sun also represents **attention-seeking** or **status-conveying items and purchases, such as flashy cars or show homes (KW, QW, 10P).**

A note of caution: all your financial dealings are likely to become public knowledge when this card appears, though this may be done intentionally to attract admiration or attention (Lovers) or for some more underhanded purpose (Devil). When flanked by negative cards, the Sun can indicate **wealth or status (Emperor, Empress, KW, QW)** being utilized as a beacon to attract or control others (Devil). The Sun energy can **attract the wrong type of attention** and inadvertently alienate others by being overly **flashy, showy or boasting of their wealth and success (Devil, KW, QW)**.

Also, unless carefully scrutinized (KS, QS, KnS) during periods of low self-esteem (Moon), the **'Because I'm worthy' attitude to purchasing only serves to temporarily pump up a punctured ego.**

Health and Well-being

The Sun archetype in a reading is **the proverbial 'picture of health'**. It indicates a healthy and well-functioning heart, for **just as the Sun radiates life-giving energy to the solar system, so the heart circulates blood, oxygen, warmth, nutrients and life to the body.**

The Sun also signifies **excellent health and a great feeling of well-being instilled via a deep sense of self-worth and social security. The Sun's warmth imbues us with the vitality, energy, stamina, personal confidence, courage, optimism, belief and authority necessary to sustain a public, active, driven, outgoing or high-energy role in life. This card, therefore, indicates a summer trip or holiday, perhaps in the southern hemisphere, the equatorial areas of the world or travelling in an east to west direction.**

Any problems indicated by negatively toned surrounding cards could pertain to **eyesight, the chest, and over-exposure in** the form of sunburn, as well as burning skin conditions or irritations.

The Sun also indicates **absolute purists with strong personal opinions about what should or shouldn't be consumed.** Though balanced attention to diet (Temperance) can have **great and positive health benefits,** when our personal consumption becomes a control-based obsession (Devil), these benefits can come at the expense of our greater psychological well-being.

20 JUDGEMENT XX

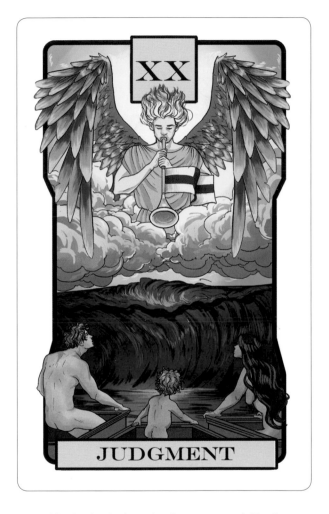

'I suddenly think the job of acting is a difficult one.
It's not as flip, irrelevant and shallow a calling as
I thought it was in the Eighties.'

ROWAN ATKINSON

Personification – Psychology

The Judgement archetype symbolizes **crossing a threshold from one phase of life to the next after a major life review**. It is the moment of **integrating all our important life lessons,** a moment of committing to **a more principled and divinely aligned life, dedicated to the betterment of ourselves and others.** The psychology of Judgement is one of ultimate **responsibility for our previous actions, the initial moment of self-realization and spiritual awakening** that eventually frees us completely (World) from an otherwise ignorant life.

The Judgement card signifies **the end of an old cerebral cycle** whereby we, having completely relinquished any old, obsolete, redundant aspects of the Self (Tower, 10S), can **ready ourselves for a new chapter.** This is the moment **we prepare to rise again,** perhaps after a fall of some kind (Tower, Death), **having integrated the hardest lessons of the previous cycle's instruction.**

When Judgement appears, our social and/or professional sense of self is primed to undergo a **sudden rebirth, regrowth, renewal, reanimation, regeneration, rejuvenation, resurgence, reinstating, realignment, reconnection, reorientation, resurrection, resuscitation, redefinition, reconstruction, reconnection, revitalization, renaissance, reinvention, reaffirmation, reactivation and recovery.**

This **radical change** is made possible only after the destruction (Death, Tower, 10S) and **removal of the veils of delusion** (Moon) that previously obscured our core self as a keeper of the deeper mysteries of life and the universe (Star). This **cerebral rebirth is akin to a crab outgrowing and shedding its shell or a snake its skin (Tower, 10S).** It is an **en-lightening process** whereby **the conscious aspect of the mind, or soul, breaks through the ego and exposes the mind to a greater intensity of**

divine light. After many cycles of expansion, the peak of this process can be seen in the symbol of the golden halo found around the heads of saintly figures in sacred works of art.

While some voluntarily welcome this period of **rebirth**, others are driven to it as a final survivalist strategy when the toxic load (10W) of emotions accumulated during the previous cycles desperately needs to be offloaded (10S). Everyone has **a restless urge toward self-reinvention,** but whether we welcome and facilitate it or create suffering for ourselves by resisting it is what makes human psychology so complex.

After huge or repeated blasts to our defensive ego-shielding (Tower, 10S), forgiving those who have wronged us is the only way to induce **deep and transformative rebirth. Then we can finally detach from all our previously intoxicating ideas about ourselves and our world.** Forgiveness does not excuse bad behaviour, or erase the memory of a harmful act, but rather assists in **detoxifying the assaulted ego, which has intensified our pain and suffering (Moon).** As prescribed by the thirteenth-century Italian Saint Francis of Assisi, '**It is in pardoning that we are pardoned.**'

The skilfulness of the Judgement archetype is in **the cultivation of an automatic and immediate tendency towards forgiveness.** It encourages viewing others' offensive behaviour as being of their own making, not ours, and so we disown this negative energy and return it forthwith to the sender. **This is what is meant by for-giveness: to give forth or back.**

Embracing this archetypal Judgement energy **can spark an all-encompassing forgiveness campaign, where we absolve all those who have ever intentionally or unintentionally hurt us.** Only then, when we have offloaded our negativity, can we again be wholly healed and free (World).

Spirituality and Philosophy

Judgement's psychic-initiation process determines whether our previous self-awakening or self-realization efforts are worthy of a higher, more en-lightened level of consciousness (Sun, Magician, High Priestess). It assesses whether we have cultivated the necessary level of indifference to the dualistic up–down, love–hate, joy–pain cycles of our earthly existence (Wheel of Fortune), or whether we still reactively resist them.

When Judgement appears, the faults in our sleepwalking ego self are exposed to be judged. No matter who has helped expose our faults, the considerable boost they have given to our conscious awareness allows us to forgive them utterly and completely. Judgement allows us to understand how the hurtful and cutting words (KS, QS, KnS) of our perceived 'enemies' called attention to our spiritual blocks, so they could be processed and overcome (1S, 1W, 1C). This is the beauty of the Judgement archetype, not only revealing the authentic, divine self, but also the myriad spiritual blessings the ignorant mind worked overtime to conceal and disguise.

This archetype helps us look back and realize that what we thought were terrible times were actually the most spiritually rewarding of our lives. Its disenchanting filter then rejects and replaces our previous identity, refining the cognitive mind so it can facilitate ever-greater spiritual realizations (High Priestess, 1C).

Personal Life

Judgement indicates **the final resolution of a relationship question that has long gone unanswered.** Perhaps after a protracted period of doubt and uncertainty (Moon), **a final decision has been reached: to continue or end a significant relationship.**

This is **the final 'clarion call' for complete honesty (KS, QS) in emotional relationships (2C, Lovers),** which could bring the great realization that something fundamental is missing (8C), or that you and your partner don't share the same values, goals, dreams, wishes and trajectory in life (2S).

Equally, a relationship that you thought was over (Death, Tower, 5C, 3S), could, via **a major release of past hurts and grievances, be resurrected, resuscitated and reborn (Aces).** Judgement can indicate the sort of **conscious relationship** where both partners realize that their judgements and values are theirs alone, and therefore cease to project them onto their counterpart. When this happens, a couple is completely **freed from the conflict and criticism** that were brandished at heated points in their relationship (5W). Being **on the edge of losing each other for good** can, when handled well, take a relationship dynamic far beyond the previous status quo (1C, 2C, 10C). However, this major archetypical release-settlement can also signal **the final cutting of your emotional attachment to each other.**

Judgement signifies **a time of forgiveness, which facilitates moving on after severe hurt or conflict in a relationship.** This **huge effort to forgive and release the past** works not only as a **survival strategy** for life, but also in committed relationships and marriage. By **forgiving truly, deeply and completely,** we reopen and drop the guard around our heart, so we are able to reaffirm our love and relationship commitment.

The archetypical swift conclusion of the Judgement card signifies a greater level of cooperation, either with your higher,
guiding self and/or with another person, if your most authentic
and genuine paths to happiness are aligned (8W).

Professional Life

Judgement indicates the make or break moment, the last word,
the major overview, review, verdict or judgement of your work or
study efforts (8P); the moment when a product, project or proposal gets the go-ahead to move forward or is permanently put
to bed – which it is depends on the tone of the outcome card.

This is likely to be the absolute or final conclusion of a major
or epic work question, the final clarification on the right path to
take or move to make, that sets our professional trajectory for
the foreseeable future.

As the agent of big revelations, the Judgement archetype helps
us finally realize our true calling in life, and thus provides the
strong internal or interior drive, impulse, purpose, reason and
directive (Moon) that is needed to propel us forward.

This card indicates the redefinition, rebirth, relaunch or reaffirmation of a product, service, idea or professional public
image, which, due to its greater authenticity and/or higher
awareness and understanding of life, will be recognized and
rewarded. Something prominent which has fallen into obscurity
is likely to be making a major comeback. Judgement reinvents,
redefines and reinterprets what once was, rendering it more
pleasing, accessible and applicable to the modern era and contemporary sensibilities. So something is about to have its
moment in the spotlight again, yet it has transformed into a far
better version of itself, with more to offer its audience, and even
perhaps humanity.

Judgement is **the pinnacle of learning via the integration of directly experienced wisdom lessons.** There is **a distinct improving quality to the work** associated with this card, either in the theme or substance of a product, project or service.

At its best, Judgement presents **a final solution, so a major ongoing problem or frustration can be rightly resolved.**

Property – Finances – Resources

The Judgement impetus for a **liberating identity change** can, when surrounded by cards indicating material comfort or luxury living standards (Empress, (9P, 10P), be **abundantly transformative on a material level.** It could be that **a life-changing financial sum** from a windfall or inheritance (10P) is on its way. Equally, you could be **reaffirming a major business or legal contract (Justice).**

This card is a fair indication of **buying up (1P), selling up (10P) or borrowing a significant sum of money (6P).** It can be **the final selling or buying of a long-term home (4W),** or receiving **a final pay cheque** from an employer and perhaps using it to launch, or relaunch, a business of your own (1W, 1P).

Conversely, it may also indicate **the final collapse of a business (Tower, Death), the final call for bank loans or any other forms of credit to be paid (5P) or the final letting go of all that you have amassed or acquired financially and/or materially (Fool).**

Health and Well-being

With this archetype in a health reading, you can experience a second lease of life after any debilitating health challenges. But it can also signify the final acceptance or realization that your poor lifestyle choices cannot continue, perhaps after the shocking results (Tower) of a health evaluation or medical review (7P).

Higher Judgement inspires the initiation of a new (Aces) health, well-being or exercise regime and the final tempering or quitting of vices (Temperance): drinking, smoking, overeating, undereating or any other unhealthily addictive predilection.

The major rebirth indicated by this archetype could be physically as well as psychologically transformative, if, for instance, you are having major surgery, especially cosmetic surgery, or experiencing bodily changes induced via hormonal replacement or any other intensive therapy. Even if you experience a physical change, due to the mind–body complex, the loss of that defining attribute of your bodily appearance can have an equal and simultaneous effect on your character or ego personality.

Whatever it is, with this card, something that you had previously been unhealthily attached to is likely to become part of Judgement's physical or emotional release settlement.

Thus, when this card appears, you are ready to rise up and let go of whatever is blocking or restricting you, whether it be on a spiritual, emotional, material or physical level, for all are inextricably synched.

21 THE WORLD XXI

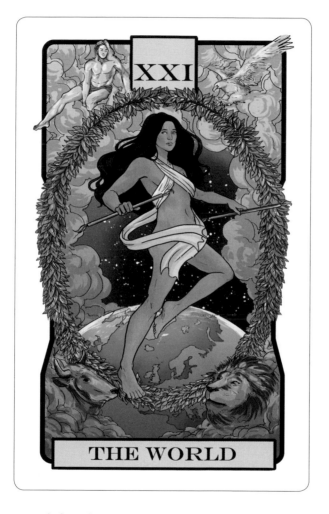

'Each friend represents a world in us . . . and it is
only by [our] meeting that a new world is born.'
ANAÏS NIN

Personification – Psychology

As the final card in the Major Arcana, the World signifies a moment of self-actualization, when all our life lessons and all disparate aspects of our being have been reintegrated, rendering our psyche complete, whole: holy. It indicates the deepest possible level of fulfilment and satisfaction, born of a sense that we have finally realized our fullest potential in life. The fullest, most authentic expression of ourselves is finally having its moment.

For the single reason that it attributes great meaning and purpose to our life, the World is the most life-affirming card in the deck. This is the peak moment in our psychological development, when all the plot threads of life come together and reveal the beautiful intricacy of its greater design.

Our unique and personal soul-expression, whatever that may be, is now wholly and openly received. We are reaching out beyond the boundaries of our own life to touch and imprint the lives of others. A desire we may have harboured or nurtured since our idealistic student days now has a voice, platform and expression to help evolve and transform society.

From our beginning as a young, idealistic Fool, we have now reached the end of our developmental journey and become a holistically synthesized, astute and Worldly being. Most striking about this is coming full circle in terms of a renewed appreciation of life. Suddenly we see everything afresh and intensely, as if for the first time, through innocent, childlike eyes (6C) that are working alongside our Worldly mind.

Reaching the point of the fullest possible self-actualization denoted by the World archetype is rare, even though, in the view of organismic theorist Kurt Goldstein, the human organism has but one basic drive and master motive: 'to actualize itself as fully as possible'. Often our lives are full of compromise, or our higher dreams and ambitions placed behind practical concerns or needs. This archetype indicates that all our basic wants and needs, on a mental, emotional, physical and spiritual level, are being met via **the full expression of our greatest individual potential and personal capacity (Sun).**

What constitutes **Worldly fulfilment** will vary from one individual to the next. For some, greater self-esteem can supersede the desire for an unhealthy love addiction, or a creative or inventive project can surpass the desire for the usual, socially expected upgrade of our basic survival needs. One individual may desire to be a loved and cherished parent, while another may find their **wholeness and completion** in reaching the peak of an athletic, musical or dramatic expression. Whatever they are, our Worldly drives, impulses and ambitions are the vital force that determines the course of our entire life.

The World's view of life is **expansive, optimistic and positive**, and thus this archetype **motivates us to realize our fullest potential.** It stands in stark contrast to the limited view that we are and will remain a product of our conditioning. The World, by its very nature, **moves us beyond our personal barriers, pushing our boundaries and widening our horizons.**

The World archetype symbolizes **the blossoming of the growth-motivated seed planted in our mind at birth.** The seed has always carried the potential for our self-actualization; in the cerebral conditions of the World, it has finally found the solid ground in which to root and fruit again.

There is a feeling of having **reached the summit, the pinnacle, the peak of existence;** to be **living as a fully functioning and optimized human being,** having overcome any culturally conditioned and disruptive forms of behaviour that have convoluted the workings of an otherwise ordered and efficient life.

The natural attributes of **a Worldly, self-actualized mentality are: feeling fully and completely ourselves, a fully functioning** human; feeling completely alive and fulfilled (wanting for nothing); being able to be completely vulnerable and risk everything at any moment, as if we had nothing to lose and everything to gain; completely integrating any painful shadow aspects, letting our higher mind heed our every word and action.

In addition, the Worldly mentality has a self-deprecating sense of humour and the ability to laugh at itself, and it is comfortable, tolerant and accepting of its own and others' flaws, shortcomings or contradictory ways of being, all of which are viewed kindly and compassionately, as part of our natural human mandate.

Whether you are well or moderately educated, rich or poor, famous or unknown, the Worldly mentality is available and accessible to you.

Spirituality and Philosophy

Each character in the tarot's sequential Major Arcana personifies the process of our ego dross transmuting into an imperishably pure golden consciousness via the reconciliation of these diametrical differences. Being the final card in the sequence, the World symbolizes the peak of this alchemical process, when we have integrated all the lessons of the Major Arcana and can, once again, embody the care-freed attitude of a hindsighted Fool.

The World archetype indicates the attainment of a state of consciousness in which we experience a union with the ultimate source of reality, the supreme being/universal architect: God. This is the pinnacle of self-realization, the end of our quest for spiritual enlightenment.

It is a universal process: the 'beingness', 'awareness' and 'meaningful happiness' of western theories on self-actualization bear a striking resemblance to the **eastern wisdom teachings on self-transcendence, where 'being'** (*sat*), **'consciousness'** (*chit*) and **'bliss'** (*ananda*) **are the peak formation of humanistic thinking and experience.**

When our surfaced soul alchemically ascends from the body, the physical, earth and water plane of our being, it returns again to its elemental home in the air. This gives the complete freedom to return to the soul plane, sometimes called **the 'out-of-body' state, which is the final spirit level of ascendence.** This is **the stuff our more lucidly spiritualized dreams are made of, a more complete picture of our three-dimensionally fragmented extra-sensory perceptions.**

The Worldly mind, being **sensitive to the fake or inauthentic, judges all situations accurately and honestly.** Its all-seeing perception allows us to move beyond mundane concerns and view reality 'as it is'. Our core self, freed from the encumbering layers of the lower-minded ego personality, can now see through (High Priestess, Sun) and wholly disengage from all mundane Earth-plane dramas.

Personal Life

If the World appears in a reading, your interpersonal relationships at this time are likely to be **profoundly true and loving (2C), marked by the deepest possible bond and the reconciliation of your individual beliefs or world views with those of a partner (10C).**

Whether in a couple or single, your manner of relating has **transcended any limiting co-dependencies.** You now feel **interdependently reliant on your own experiences to form your opinions, views and judgements.** This is a manner of relating where you are **wholly and completely true to yourself, rather than** responsively being or acting in line with how others untruly see you (Moon, Devil, 7C). Marked by a natural free-spirited spontaneity and assured sense of autonomy, the Worldly relationship is not reliant on external authorities for views on who or how to love.

If you are single, this card can denote meeting someone who makes you feel whole, who brings you out in some way, and reveals and celebrates your truest self and potential (Sun).

The new world you encounter via a relationship could literally be a foreign country, as this archetype can also signify an overseas or foreign affair, travelling with a romantic partner (Lovers) or meeting an exotic new love interest (1C) on your travels (Chariot, KnW). This is likely to be someone similarly regulated by an expansive personal campaign of tolerance and approval of diversity and who wholly accepts and supports your paradigmatic worldview, even if it is diametrically different from their own.

Professional Life

Working for worldwide or global organizations; working abroad; travelling with your work (KnW); international studies, worldly teachers or mentors; and receiving a world-class education (Hierophant) all fall into the sphere of this outgoing and expansive archetype.

The World presents itself when you are using all of your creative potential to fulfil the mission of your life. This could be a humanitarian problem that lies 'beyond' rather than just outside yourself, for the World archetype represents a great moment of personal fulfilment that often, but not always, has far-reaching effects or implications. It could also be a world-class service, project, idea or operation that captures the public (Sun) mood or imagination (Moon) and reflects or projects a global mood and trend (Moon).

The World archetype can signify the major manifestation (Magician) of **a trending world vision**. You may establish an excellent international reputation and world-wide following, become a world authority on your subject (Emperor, Empress, Hierophant) or receive major international recognition or validation of your skills and abilities (3P, 9C).

This is likely to be **a climactic moment for your business or career**: the perfect time to launch a new (1W, 1P) international service, project or product onto **the world stage**. The World indicates it will meet with **the widest possible recognition and success**.

Property – Finances – Resources

When this archetype is present, your project, product or service is likely to achieve **a world-ranking sales position**, with the potential for huge returns (10P), far exceeding the original time, money or energy invested. It is likely **your material assets are expanding (KP, QP, 10P)**, and this card offers **the potential to build a world-class empire (Emperor, Empress)**.

Any new sources of income (1P) are likely to appear from **much further afield, possibly as global economic forces** produce a spike (1P), or even downturn (5P), in economic income, revenue, net profit, stock and share prices. The World can indicate **money coming from foreign investments, global markets, stock trades and exchanges (2P), and international banking, trade and investment (6P)**.

The World also indicates the **buying or selling of the worldwide rights to an idea or product (1P, 3W)**. Other big purchases could include **foreign land and property**, allowing you to move abroad (4W) and significantly better your quality of life (9P, 10P, Empress).

Health and Well-being

On a mundane level, this archetype indicates a major break-through (1W, 1P, 1C) with your health and well-being. This may be due to the success of surgery (1S) or the taking of a new, improved remedy resulting in **total freedom from pain and suf-fering, or perhaps falling pregnant after many months, even years, of trying (Empress, 1C, 1W).**

Should it be needed, the World indicates that medical assist-ance can be provided (6P) by **worldly, international or internationally renowned (3P) healthcare practitioners (KC, QC), who perhaps take a holistic, foreign and exotic approach, such as physiotherapists using acupuncture needles (KS, QS, 1S).**

There is **an unsurpassed curative force in the World's natural mandate for self-realization.** Once a person relinquishes the growth-stunting feeling or belief that they are, in some way, under-functioning or physically deficient, they **finally grow into who they are: the purest, healthiest and most completed version of themselves.**

In summary, the **safety and security felt when we truly accept, honour and love ourselves, just as we are, is the secret to the holistic health of our world within and without.**

THE MINOR ARCANA

The Minor Arcana cards deal with the day-to-day events set in motion by the energetic archetypes of the Major Arcana. The fifty-six cards are divided into four suits: Wands, Cups, Pentacles and Swords. They are representations of the elemental energies – fire, water, earth and air – appearing in our life as follows:

- Wands (fire): physical energy and action
- Cups (water): feelings and emotions
- Pentacles (earth): financial, material and practical concerns
- Swords (air): thought processes and intellect

These energies can either show up in our own approach to a situation or in the approach of those who are interacting with us.

THE SUIT OF WANDS

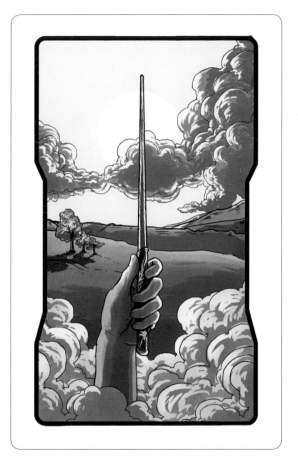

Ace of Wands

The Ace of Wands indicates that now is the time to start something new. It represents being at the beginning, being or arriving first, newness, primitiveness, primacy, priority, novelty, innovation, invention and pioneering entrepreneurship. It heralds all new forms, including the birth of a project, a child, an action and an event.

Whatever you have in mind, the time to strike is now: while the proverbial iron is hot. The Ace of Wands can feel like a sudden physical surge of energy that sets new things in motion. It can bring fresh new insight, inspiration, courage, conviction, hope, boldness, vigour, enthusiasm, vitality, creativity, mental and physical fertility.

It heralds a splendid revelation about the future, something to fill you with purpose and lighten your way in life. This could be a new direction, a new work opportunity or an innovative new product or project.

The enterprising attitude behind this Ace produces highly personalized results. It empowers us to be our completely individual selves, free of any need for validation from others.

The Ace of Wands represents our indomitable spirit of being: the enlivening, invigorating vital energy that animates all sentient life. This is the primary life-force energy, the raging internal fire, being expressed in dynamic physical actions and initiations. It represents the innate and primal forces of the human body, such as the drive to procreate, being kindled, stoked and released.

It could be that primal energies, or people who embody those energies (KW, QW, KnW, PW), suddenly appear, or reappear, bringing a new emotional surge, or the re-emergence of old feelings, invigorating a new relationship, or resurrecting an old one (Moon, 6C).

The Ace of Wands often appears when we have passed some form of initiation process, either personal, spiritual or work based, and are about to emerge or make our debut. Spiritually speaking, the Ace of Wands indicates our butterfly-like emergence from an inner process of transformation that has moved us from a 'blinkered' to eyes-wide-open existence.

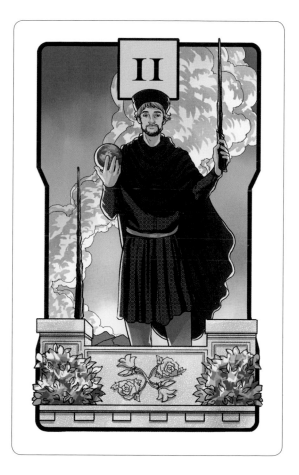

Two of Wands

The Two of Wands represents a working union or business partnership. This can be two separate individuals or business associates coming together to work on a project, under the same banner or for the same cause. This is a symbiotic, reciprocal and co-operative, aligned, dynamic, energetic, outgoing and outward-looking partnership. Both parties are in agreement over their mutual goals, values, vision for the future and what needs to be done to move things forward and expand their scope, operation, territories or travel destinations.

This is the point where you no longer have to bear the entire burden of a project, event or undertaking on your own. The union you make with another person not only benefits you both, but your mutual endeavour is all the better for it.

This card isn't just about making one-to-one alliances, though, but also about making connections in general by widening and expanding your social or business network.

As fire begets fire, in a romance reading, the Two of Wands indicates a power coupling or relationship that actively works to empower the lives of both parties.

This card equates to double the energetic input of the Ace, but not necessarily the practical or financial resources needed to sustain a material endeavour (Pentacles), or the depth of feeling needed to feel secure in a romantic relationship (Cups). Yet the castle confinement depicted does indicate the establishment of a strong dominion-style power base that acts as a supportive source of authority and influence in your cause. The success of your initial negotiations, be they personal, political or business related, will be particularly useful in later obtaining backing from those who have the practical know-how and finances to make your plans happen (Emperor, Empress, KP, QP).

Now is a time to think bigger. Expand the reach of your endeavours beyond the castle walls (3 W). Success is but a few handshakes away.

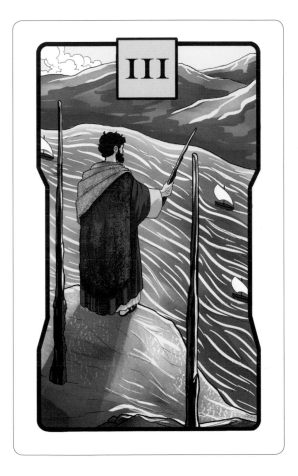

Three of Wands

The Three of Wands indicates a great sense of company, group or family loyalty, oneness, togetherness and a pack mentality. You share a vision of where you want to go in the future and are coming ever closer to making it happen. The greater power of the group is setting things in motion. Your mutual plans are expansive or travel-motivated; you move as a group in unison towards international lands or a distant future goal.

After seizing new opportunities (1W) and working with another person to build on them (2W), you see them multiply. You are now likely to be looking to the wider world of industry with a new action (1W), product (1P), concept or idea (1S). There is an indication of studying your global, international or foreign competitors (5W) before making the final move into their territory. When found in combination with certain major cards (Emperor, World), world market domination is a distinct possibility.

Whether business related or otherwise, your efforts are internationally or future focused, with far-reaching potential. The international expansion of your business is possible by establishing an international network of dynamic social or business contacts, new clients (1P) and promotional agents (KnW, 8W). The Three is a card of globalization, of thinking globally rather than locally. Making global connections and international networking (Chariot, KnW) can result in mutually lucrative international or foreign exchange deals (1P).

When this card appears, you could be making a contribution to the wider world community, a global cause, working overseas or in the travel industry (KnW), or broadening your educational horizons by taking a gap year abroad (World, KnW, KnC).

Whatever is happening, this card indicates finding a creative balance and living a future-focused life fired by work, play and a revitalized sense of your spiritual or personal calling.

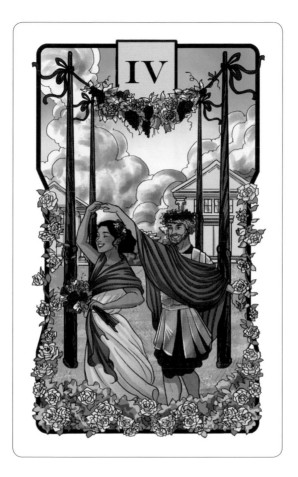

Four of Wands

The Four of Wands represents fun – life-affirming events or activities that bring joy, happiness, rejoicing and respite. These can be special occasions, celebrations, ceremonies, entertainments, amusements, main events, attractions, parties, performances, art, music, dance, drama and games. The card can indicate friendships, love, romance, birthdays, engagements, weddings or any sort of victorious or celebratory times spent with those you love or who fill you with joy.

As a card of stability (Four) in action (Wands), it can also indicate a positive and wished-for home or office move, or a relationship actively taken to the next level of commitment (2C). In a relationship reading, it could be that plans to buy a property or move in together have come to fruition.

The success of a work endeavour, creative project, business venture or big promotion could be what has instigated your move up in the world, be it literal or metaphorical. Staying in hot pursuit of your goals and ambitions, while working diligently to garner more knowledge and gain more experience, has paid off.

The Four of Wands is a card of entrepreneurial marksmanship – your financial decisions have been 'right on the money'. It indicates a certain confidence in raising capital and mobilizing money, perhaps to make future-focused investments in a creative or dynamic business venture. The solid foundations of your work life and finances will bring a greater sense of personal comfort, safety and security.

When the Four of Wands appears, there is a sense of joy and satisfaction in your accomplishments, in having reached a key milestone on the journey towards your ultimate goal (World, 10C, 10P). Now is the time to reap the rewards of your previous efforts, generosity, drive or enthusiasm, whether these have been directed towards a relationship, job, project, activity or spiritual discipline. The Force of the Wands is most definitely with you.

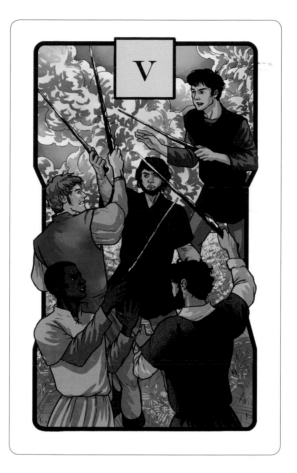

Five of Wands

The Five of Wands indicates a state of chaos driven by a battle of wills, a heated contest, complications, disputes, arguments, obstacles, opponents, conflict, enemies, fighting, challenge, combat, competition, rivalry and struggle. Tough times may be testing your self-confidence, courage and pride.

In defending or going after your goals, it's likely that you are feeling challenged or are challenging someone else. Your business, projects, products or services could be facing fierce competition in the market-place or you may have had to battle for a promotion, salary increase or new contract.

This Five indicates conflict as a result of an unconscious partnership's dysfunctional, painful and oppressive power struggles and ego battles. Being competitive could end your relationship (Death, Tower, 3S, 5C). Your work or social life could be competing with a lover/partner for your attention, or vice versa. If single, you may be facing competition for the object of your affections, or be the desired object being fought over.

This card indicates unsettled rhythms and life conditions: your body may be fighting off ill-health or an infection. Taking up a competitive team sport is a positive way to channel this frenetic energy. As long as it doesn't spring from destructive emotions, such as greed and jealousy, a little competition can keep your energy focused and your mind dynamically engaged.

This card calls your attention to the mental resistance born of unexamined ego attachments (Moon, Devil). The Five of Wands' type of pain, resulting from internal and external ego conflicts, can force us to examine, and ultimately resolve, our ingrained emotional issues.

Your spiritual belief system may also conflict with your material or physical concerns or with the beliefs of an associate or closer counterpart. Respecting each individual's beliefs and approach to life – essentially taking life more lightly, as if it were just a game being played – will help you accept any perceived loss as you would a gain. To win the game of life (6W), start by challenging your own self-concept and perception.

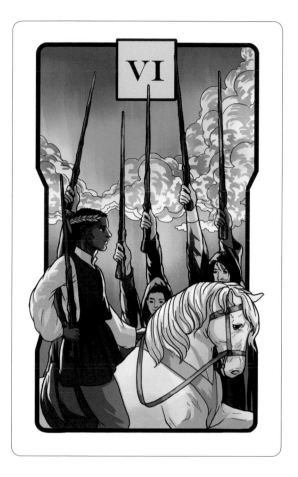

Six of Wands

The Six of Wands indicates the success of an external or internal form of conflict resolution. Only the physically, mentally, emotionally, materially strongest or fittest will have made it through the tests of the previous card (5 W); ironically, out of the chaos of that battle, you may have found an opportunity to advance your cause.

It is likely that you are jubilant and celebrating after having heard some satisfying news, something that constitutes a vindication or the realization of a hope, wish or desire. Your honour, stealth, skill, agility, timing, quick thinking and flexibility of mind and body have led you to a resounding victory.

This is a moment of garnering awards or rewards, fame and acclaim, and generally being admired for your triumphant achievements. Through unwavering hard work, drive, ambition and a strong belief in yourself and your own abilities you have overcome all obstacles and obtained a much-desired outcome.

When this card appears, any pending decisions, be they emotional, financial, work or study related, will be very much in your favour. It could be that you have received a long-awaited promotion, work contract (Justice) or pay rise (6P), or the exam results you were hoping for.

After trouble and strife in a relationship, or in finding the right partner, the Six of Wands indicates a reason to feel joyfully relieved. It could be that previous challenges and difficulties have brought you closer to a partner, helping you forge a deeper bond and re-establish a commitment.

This is a time when emotional, material and speculative financial investments, especially those that have consumed a great deal of your time and energy, are likely to be handsomely paying off or bringing in a substantial profit.

If health, fitness or general well-being have been your focus, this card heralds the rewards of a more conscious attempt to clean up and clear out your physical, mental and emotionally energetic junk, i.e. any toxic or negative thoughts or feelings that are driving your everyday actions.

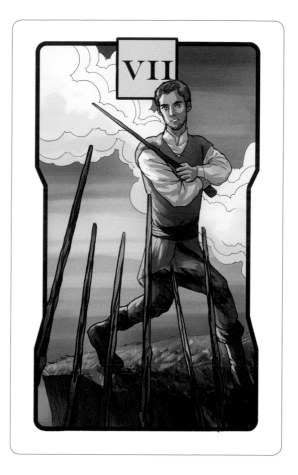

Seven of Wands

The Seven of Wands indicates being well prepared to defend your territory, beliefs or position with heroic will and determination. People may be attempting to criticize your actions, press your buttons, question your authority or the validity of your decisions. This is a life-defining moment, where you establish your core identity by rebuffing those who seek to challenge your personal worth and validity. It is the moment you stave off all those who represent your old, redundant, lower-minded fears as they try and fail to undermine the core confidence of the higher mind.

In previous cards (Hermit), we saw the unstable ego becoming consciously aware of itself for the first time – aware of the performance it was staging and the attention it needed to survive as your life's prime leader or controller. The Seven of Wands indicates that your newly stabilized ego-self is suffering an invalidation attack from those who have yet to free themselves.

The health and resilience of the ego, whether it is strong or weakened by our upbringing, is usually determined by our primary educators and care providers. The Seven of Wands indicates the health of your ego being tested by weakened ego personalities. A series of such testers may be coming into your life. They may be friends, partners, family members, work colleagues, students, teachers or anyone else who is intimately or often involved in your life. The more fragile the egos testing and challenging your stance, position or identity, the more intense, desperate, anxious, fractious and mutually exhausting their interference will be.

The Seven of Wands can be a life-defining challenge, where retaining your balance and integrity of purpose will preserve your optimal, higher or advantageous position.

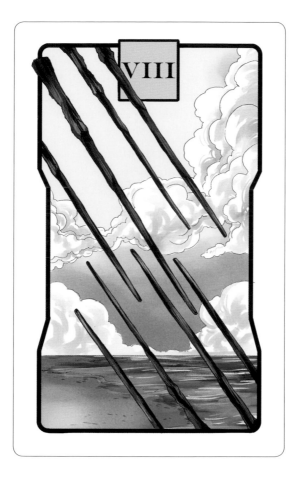

Eight of Wands

The Eight of Wands signifies a greater level of efficiency, alignment and cooperation, either with yourself or others. It represents a swift and immediate forward movement, or the sudden great release of any pent-up energy, directed towards a desired goal free of any blocks or impediments.

There is a boldness, daring, exploratory and expansive nature to this card, whether it relates to love, work, wealth or health. The direct energy behind your motivations and agenda is clean, clear and aligned with your true interests. This card is, therefore, referred to as the arrows of love, as it indicates two people's paths being truly and harmoniously aligned, rather than crossing over, impeding or convoluting the directional flow of each other's energy or journey.

The Eight of Wands represents big revelations and all forms of communication or communicative action (Sun). This could be your words being read or voice being heard (Sun, KS, QS), you being seen (Sun, KW, QW), a new promotion or product launch taking place (1W, 1P, 1C), feelings being felt or shared (KC, QC), or the joyful announcement of a marriage (4W), engagement (3C) or pregnancy (Empress, 1W, 1C, 1P).

The card also symbolizes satellite-linked computer or phone connectivity (Star); the internet and online endeavours; TV, radio, news transmissions or broadcasting (8W, Sun); global PR and marketing campaigns; and tapping into what is current, of the moment or mainstream (Sun).

This is a card of contemporary ideas being widely shared and how news of these travels hyper fast to established new paradigms overnight. It indicates major personal or emotional (Cups), professional, financial, social, cultural, political and institutional momentum. Events could progress very quickly and efficiently.

Overall, this is a card of swift, conclusive, resolute decisions sweeping aside past doubt, uncertainty, ambiguity, impediments, obfuscations (Moon), obstructions (5W) and delays (8S) to move things swiftly forward.

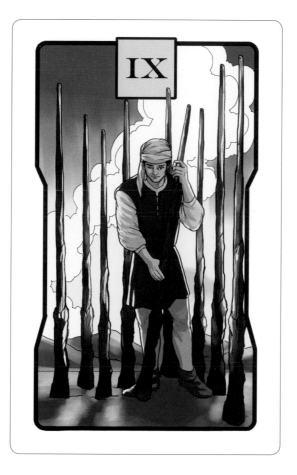

Nine of Wands

This card represents all forms of compartmentalizing and self-defence and protectionism (Moon), whether physical (Wands), intellectual (Swords), emotional (Cups) or material (Pentacles).

In a relationship, it indicates trust issues, when you become overly self-protective and invulnerable, leaving no room for closeness or intimacy. Fear-based decisions and actions (Moon, 8S, 9S) taken to try to protect yourself from further pain and suffering will only backfire.

Mentally, the Nine of Wands indicates storage of and resistance to any offences committed against you. But the fuller the hard drive of your mind becomes, the slower and more inefficient its functioning.

Also, when the mind expends a great deal of energy resisting, we reap a great deal more negativity from a situation. Any situation becomes more difficult as a consequence of active resistance to it. Our thoughts can make the experience worse than it need actually be by allowing a past or reimagined fear of being hurt to engage our emotional defence mechanism (Moon), which negatively affects our mood and temperament.

As a symbol of the wounded ego protecting the most vulnerable aspects of the self, the Nine of Wands stands together as the individual scaffolding of our core identity. This scaffolding is constructed of our self-justifications and entitlements, established by our carers and educators to stabilize and place us in the world. This leads us to believe that our way of operating, whether morally, emotionally or materially, is *the* way.

The Nine of Wands often turns up in a reading when the characteristic attributes of another person's ego-scaffolding conflict with our own, leaving us feeling we must defend our belief system or lose our true, authentic sense of self in the process. However, this is purely an illusion or trick of the ego-powered mind; when a negative, invalidating energy attempts an attack, a healthy and mindful and conscious person can easily withstand it.

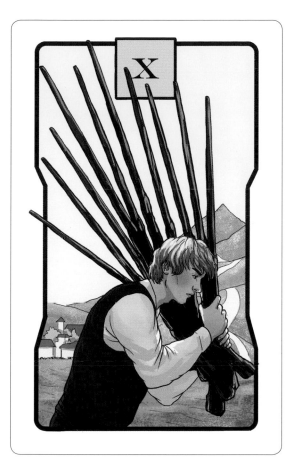

Ten of Wands

This can be a time of charismatic overreaching or overextending, being overworked or voluntarily becoming a workaholic. There can be an amplification of ambition to reach political, theatrical, glamorous or creative goals, which may even include childbearing or pregnancy (Sun).

Comforting habits (Moon) or other forms of stress release

may now be prevented by onerous duties, heavy obligations, intensity of pressure and feeling overburdened, perhaps due to a lack of support (Hermit, 5P). The Ten indicates extremely hard work for which you sacrifice freedom, leisure or pleasure, but usually for what you consider to be a worthwhile cause.

You may, however, be trying too hard and spreading yourself thinly. The many commitments you have taken on in life, love and work are slowing your overall progress. Tiredness and fatigue are likely to be brought on by this increased workload or these heavier responsibilities, with no assistance from others. This is a greater burden than you can carry alone; delegating some responsibility to others will ease the process. Efficiency and ergonomics of movement and action are key to the health and well-being of not only your bodily posture, but also your property, wealth and finances.

You may feel your accomplishments are lacking praise or credit from others, or feeling socio-cultural pressure, either from your family or the wider community, to keep within the bounds of convention (Hierophant).

Certainly the Ten of Wands indicates a time when hard work or study are the primary source of your core validation. Relationships can be held back now, either by heavy work obligations or the cumulatively toxic effect of holding on to the sadness, anger and humiliation amassed during any previous identity conflict with others (5W). By holding on to anger and resentment, though, you find the journey of life is burdened and impeded by the psychic weight of your internal suffering. Only complete forgiveness will set you free (Judgement).

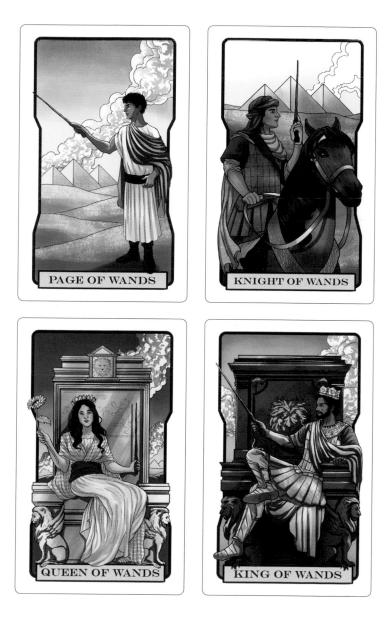

Wands Court Cards

The Wands courtiers are energetic representations of fire energy at work in our life – or, perhaps, we are working it. All the court cards share the elemental motivations, agendas, desires and impulses pertaining to the ruling element of the suit to which they belong, but how each of the courtiers applies themselves to a situation depends on their individual level of development and maturity. The Wands courtiers are: the Page (PW), an immature or underdeveloped male or female energy or personality; the Knight (KnW), a moving-towards and outgoing male or female energy or personality; the Queen (QW) and King (KW), fully developed, realized, mature and established female and male energies or personalities.

The first plane of our alchemical human being is fire, the primordial element represented by the suit of Wands, which transmutes and transforms the physical, bodily planes of earth and water, creatively bringing them into being, through myriad objects, shapes and forms.

As representatives of the fire element, the Wands courtiers are individual and different, with great imaginative vision, creative intelligence and integrity of purpose. They boldly take on challenges that others might consider terrifying or insurmountable. These courtiers know that how full and expansive their lives are correlates directly to their level of personal assertiveness, daring and courage. Their showy, dramatic or theatrically staged 'reasoning' can be time-wasting when a practical, articulate or logically valid argument needs to be made. However, their potential for characterful, expressive and engaging output is key for public speakers, commercial writers, entertainers, actors or performers.

As highly charismatic, vivacious, physically magnetic personalities, the Wands courtiers are prone to flagrant self-glorification, excessive self-promotion and boasting of their projected success on public forums and social media sites such as 'Brag Book'. But, rather than bringing them the love they seek, these actions can tend to alienate or isolate them from those they would most like to impress.

Whether real or imagined (Moon, 7C), any fame, celebrity or notoriety they acquire tends to reduce the circle of friends they can really trust – those who like them for who they really are beneath the bright and sparkling public projection. By projecting an image of themselves as a great or significant person, the King and Queen of Wands are often left yearning for the intimate company of true friends rather than their distant, artificial admirers. The great life lesson for the Wands courtiers is to overcome their need for the attention, adoration and approval of others (Moon).

This idea is evoked in the Greek myth of the young Icarus (PW), who, ignoring his father's logical instruction (KS), impetuously took to the air with a set of wings made from feathers and wax and shortly afterwards plummeted to his death when the was melted from the heat of the Sun (the fame and glory he sought). Pride coming before a fall has been repeated in many a moralistic allegory or fable and tends to be the story behind all of the Wand courtiers' greatest mistakes.

In their glorified position this suit can also sometimes lack sympathy or empathy for those weaker or more vulnerable than themselves and must guard against being overly self-righteous, smug, hubristic, pompous, conceited, pretentious, proud, arrogant, superior, patronizing, self-involved, self-absorbed, solipsistic, self-reflexive, demanding, brash, hurried, impatient, rash, strident, forceful, pushy, slapdash and impetuous.

However, the heated energy of these courtiers is useful in all situations requiring a forceful, belligerent, bold, impulsive, impatient, confident, courageous, daring, determined, aspiring, ambitious, goal-oriented, energetic, manifesting, emergent (Aces) or urgent approach.

The Wands courtiers represent people and situations that are competitive (5W), masculine, outgoing, energetic, active, purposeful, pursuing, dominating, supreme, powerful, strong, defensive and forceful, often involving fast-acting, 'hungry' individuals in 'hot' pursuit of something or someone (KnW). They are actors, agents, seekers, searchers, hunters, movers and shakers (KW, QW), leaders or even just figureheads of the business, political, creative and theatrical worlds.

The Knight, in particular, can be the international face of a business or in a job involving a fair amount of international travel (KnW). The exploratory Wands courtiers often take a broad overview of a situation before pursuing their goals and ambitions with great vigour, intensity, confidence and determination.

Embodying the enlivening life-force energy that animates all sentient life, the Wands courtiers are the vital and indomitable spirit behind our very being, and as such feel constrained, impeded and restless when pitted against slower-moving (Hermit) or socially and culturally constrictive cards (Hierophant). Their energy allies with all cards that are boundlessly active (Fool), fast-moving or energetically outgoing (Sun, Wands, Swords); their inner engine is stoked by those people or places that, like themselves, have a raging internal fire.

The Wands courtiers' self-concept is one of the inherently able and capable executive, athlete, fighter, competitor, warrior, champion and best in the field, or a closely ranked associate of other highly placed or visible people (Sun, Empress, High Priestess, Hierophant). Due to their naturally outgoing and assertive personality, their point of view is rarely hidden unless there are any covert influences (High Priestess, Moon, Devil).

They can be highly enterprising and, under the right influences, the cause or initiator of great positive or benevolent (High Priestess, Temperance, KC, QC), pure and noble-hearted actions

(Strength, Temperance, Sun). However, under destructive (Tower, Death) or ego-inflating influences (Devil), the negatively impassioned Wands courtier can be rash, aggressive, impulsive, jealous, violent (5W) or easily led astray (Fool).

The King and Queen of Wands can be supremely confident and pioneering in the arenas of politics, speculations, games, the procreation of children, the performing or creative arts, fashion, celebrity, royalty, romance, glamour and charisma (Sun).

As leaders, politicians, trendsetters, fashionistas, performers and actors, the Wands courtiers, no matter what their gender, can be hot-headed, self-important or self-dramatizing personalities. Their core certainty makes no allowance for shyness, confusion, doubt, uncertainty, fear or ambiguity (Moon), and they don't work well with those who lack purpose or conviction.

When the Wands courtiers appear in a reading, you may be feeling eclipsed or subjugated by those who are more highly placed or visibly positioned than you are.

When their radiant exterior is diminished or eclipsed by a brighter flame, perhaps from someone who possesses a desired but under-represented quality in themselves, the insecure Wands courtier may try to darken or completely extinguish this perceived threat. Whether they are a company manager (KW) or a proverbial socialite 'Queen Bee' (QW), they often go to great lengths to chop off the top of the taller-standing tree. Being victimized in this way, or inadvertently deemed worthy via the attack, paradoxically proves your greater worth.

At their very worst (Devil), the Wands courtiers can represent egoistic power-trippers or predatory narcissists who abuse their authority or perceived 'stardom'. As they lead such highly public lives, their transgressions are often found out, inducing a newsworthy fall from grace (Tower).

Conversely, when regulated and shaped by morally sound influences (Hierophant, Hermit, Justice), the primary life-force energy of the Wands can be expressed in a way that seeks to enforce or reinforce already existing laws, rules, structures and systems, and, as such, represents police, military, army, emergency, rescue or other frontline service requiring high energetic output: 'manly' (KW) or 'womanly' (QW) heroics.

The Wands courtiers are instinctive, animalistic, alive, vigorous, vital, excitable, dynamic, reactive, direct, aggressive, intense, forcible, invasive, challenging, competitive, battling, pursuant, fighting, hunting, dominating, pioneering, innovative, exploring, sporting and sexually alert. They are the singularly focused and goal-oriented movers, shakers and activators behind all causes seeking publicity and recognition, people whose work requires great physical vitality, dominant 'alpha' conqueror or animalistic-attack type instincts. In the heated pursuit of their primary goals, ambitions and causes, they can be uncompromising to the point of sacrificing everything. Surrounding cards can provide more on the motives, agenda and style of that pursuit.

In terms of health and well-being, the Wands courtiers must watch for physical irritations, excess movement, overheating, loss of fluids and dehydration. When anger and frustration arise, any vigorous and heat-releasing cardiovascular movement such as dance, running, working out, dynamic yoga, cycling, team sports or martial arts will help keep the heart, mind and energetic system functioning purely and cleanly.

THE SUIT OF CUPS

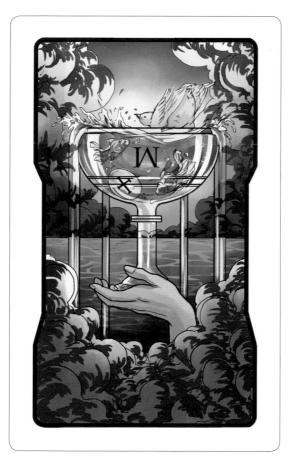

Ace of Cups

The Ace of Cups presents a new opportunity for joy, love, emotional connection, contentment, fertility, pregnancy, growth or spiritual awakening.

The overflowing Cup provides us with a vivid sense of the

subtle, unseen or spiritual realities. This card requires something deep within us to be enlivened or awakened; should it remain unconscious, we will be prevented from gaining the necessary understanding of our life purpose.

The Ace of Cups is a blessing for those who want to truly understand the spirituality of life, for which our normal, 'common sense' consciousness is inadequate. We can only truly understand another person or situation when we subjectively feel and engage, rather than objectively perceive and disengage (Pentacles). By consciously rejecting our objectively detached stance in favour of the Ace of Cup's interior intelligence, we find situations becoming deeper, more penetrative, meaningful and heartfelt.

This card, therefore, indicates all pure, heart-centred words, deeds, actions and connections, and unexpected meetings or messages concerning the same. If it appears in a reading, something you have done or produced may have moved someone to their very core or helped open their heart to you or your own heartfelt endeavours. The key to success is being completely free, open, revealing and honest, perhaps revealing truths that would otherwise have remained hidden.

Events now feel like a spiritual blessing, which brings even more grace and understanding to your handling of life's affairs (Strength).

Ultimately, the Ace of Cups can assist you in going beyond all distinctions between subject and object and enjoying a non-dualistic consciousness; transcending the self through mystical absorption, immersion, unification and at-one-ment with the universe or Absolute (High Priestess).

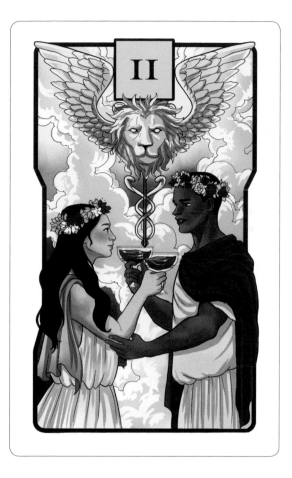

Two of Cups

The Two of Cups indicates a perfectly balanced and harmonious pairing or partnership, either in business, friendship or romance. Your deep and strong emotional connection ensures that you understand and respect each other's point of view, whether or not it is in concordance with your own.

By bringing together the diametrically different male and

female aspects, this card speaks of the natural attraction of opposites or creatively opposing forces. The answer to your question or situation may be neither black nor white, but one of the many combined shades in between.

The Two of Cups denotes a truly supportive and intimately connected partnership that helps you remain clear about what you want from life. When compromises have to be made, you make them willingly and happily when this card is present.

Whether this indicates a pledge of fidelity, an engagement (3C), marriage (Justice, 4W) or a business merger, the decision to deepen a commitment brings great love, joy, happiness and contentment to all.

You may have met a kindred spirit, someone whose presence helps you approach life and love with greater balance, peace and equanimity. This pure, sacred, heart-to-heart connection exists only on a higher, subtle and logically inexplicable plane; it can't be rationalized or quantified.

Materially speaking, the Two of Cups indicates that a partnership of some kind will increase your wealth or balance your finances. By partnering with a person who possesses the exact attributes you lack, and vice versa, you are propelled forward as half of a more complete and unified whole.

The emotional balance and equanimity of this card filters down through all areas of your life, health and general well-being. Any previous build-up of tension or pressure, whether physical, mental, emotional or material, should now begin to smoothly and gently unwind and be released.

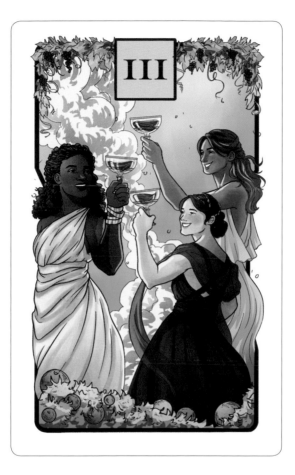

Three of Cups

The Three of Cups represents the social aspect of life: where and with whom you feel most comfortable. It is indicative of socializing, meeting new people or attending reunions with family and friends (3C), or any time when people come together to rejoice, celebrate or gather for festivities of a busy, joyous or flamboyant nature (Sun).

However, this Three, in particular, has an emotional quality, and as such the gathering depicted can be a wedding, engagement, birthday, baby shower, festival, anniversary, reunion or holiday gathering. If you are single and looking for love, this card indicates an up and coming social event worth attending.

The gathering could even be of a kindred or spiritual nature, where a diverse or unconnected group is brought together due to mutual love of or devotion to a shared cause or ideology.

Finding relief and release in dance, movement or socializing in general is strongly indicated by the Three of Cups. However, as a crossing card, indicating what is holding you back, it advises that some unhealthy social or emotional attachments (Moon) may need examining and releasing.

Music has special significance here, as the Three of Cups indicates a deep love of it and a need for it as a form of emotional release (Moon). The Three of Cups is a card of arts and creativity, such as music, theatre and performance, which all demand romantic, passionate, imaginative and fantastical (7C) inspiration.

This is a card of secure belonging, camaraderie and inclusivity, of feeling part of a closely connected group of family, friends or loved ones. As such, when it appears, former estrangements are happily mended, to the joy and relief of all.

Whether related to work, finances, romance, friends, family, health or well-being, this card signals a very happy conclusion to a heartfelt or meaningful matter.

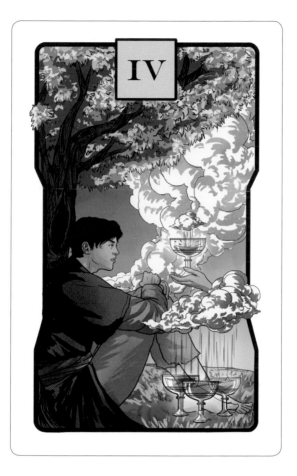

Four of Cups

The Four of Cups is a card of emotional disengagement, usually due to a deep dissatisfaction with a situation, relationship or life in general. This is a time when genuine and authentic love, affection or devotion is likely to be taken for granted. For some reason, we feel unable to show or reciprocate the love, desire, passion, enthusiasm or emotional connection that is on offer to

241

us. What is real, true and authentically felt is being ignored or considered not good enough, and what will make us happier is likely to be indefinable or inaccessible.

The lack of drive and ambition signified by the Four of Cups is coupled with a failure to recognize, appreciate or apply any real value to things, and taking life's big and small blessings continually for granted. Boredom, inertia, apathy, indifference, impartiality, dissatisfaction, disenchantment and disengagement from life and the wider world are indicated here. But emotional idleness leads only to further procrastination and stagnation (8S).

Such a lack of passion, interest and excitement with the material world may, mistakenly (Fool), be confused with spiritual truth or awakening, which, conversely, is marked by a renewed childlike engagement with all life has to offer (6C).

The Four of Cups represents the unhappy state of mind caused by self-absorption, self-involvement (Sun, KW, QW, KnW, PW) or a perpetual over-prioritization of our own personal or emotional needs above those of others (Moon). It indicates a situation limited by seeing only what we think we already know, as we select only the information that confirms our pre-existing negative or pessimistic beliefs and world view. Such low-grade thoughts and judgements, about ourselves or others, are but imagined mental constructs of 'reality' (7C).

By projecting positive and optimistic thought into the world, our mental, emotional and physical health, and even material wealth, can dramatically improve.

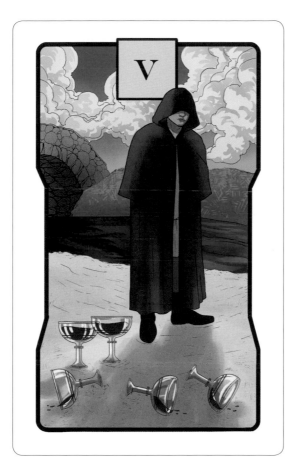

Five of Cups

The Five of Cups indicates a palpable sense of loss, grief and disappointment, where a person or situation has failed to meet your expectations. This card indicates any situation where it is hard to let go. You may be holding on to the recent or distant past, or even a past deception (Devil), looking only at what has been lost and ignoring the potential joys you still have in front of you.

This state of being left wanting, or longing for what was or might have been, brings only more suffering, sadness, grief and regret. No matter how let down you are feeling, lamenting a wrong decision, brooding over a loss or wallowing in self-pity only intensifies the pain and suffering.

This card points to unrequited love, where feelings are not reciprocated. Irreconcilable differences of character may also have led to a painful separation from an intimate companion.

In general, the Five of Cups signifies the permanent removal of our emotional support base (Hermit, Moon). In the face of such a big disappointment, where our external emotional support has been shown to be an illusion (Moon, 7C), we are prompted to find it inside ourselves (Hermit). Eliminating any non-supportive or conventionally programmed (Hierophant) emotional attachments in favour of our own self-nourishment and reliance will open us up to the possibility of healthier, inter-dependent relationships entering our life.

If a source of love and nurturing (Moon) has rejected or abandoned you, this provides the perfect opportunity to adjust your behavioural patterns, and even overhaul your search criteria. Only when you truly stop looking for what you have lost can you break the habit of forming insecure and unworthy attachments. By changing the trajectory of your thinking from past to future, you will allow a deeper and more authentic love connection to form, with yourself and others.

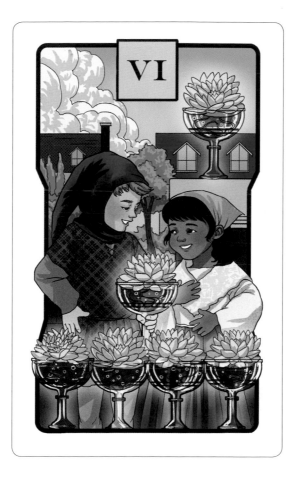

Six of Cups

The Six of Cups represents a renewed appreciation of life. Suddenly we see everything afresh and intensely, as if for the first time, with pure, innocent and honest eyes: the all-seeing eyes of an artist or a child. Such a playfully childlike world view is of great use in all the creative industries: adults often find a young child's clear, honest, straightforward, uncomplicated speech, thoughts and ideas refreshing, inspiring, endearing, entertaining and amusing, like those of a comedian who freely and easily speaks out about controversial matters.

The Six of Cups indicates our adoption of a young child's easy and carefree attitude so as to unconditionally accept the world exactly as we find it, without resistance, opposition, complication, convolution, pride, pretence, prejudice, preconception, prejudgement, predisposition, partiality, bias, bigotry, narrow-mindedness, discrimination, intolerance, injustice or partisan leanings.

This is a card of natural inclusivity, bonding and friendliness, which come from our innate inner-child sense of security and allow us to be completely open, engaged and vulnerable with others, no matter how outwardly different those others may be. This is a card where external factors have no sway or influence; the connection is emotional or spiritual, and so reaches deep beyond superficial or surface matters.

In any relationship question, this card indicates an ability to form a strong bond by allowing ourselves to be completely vulnerable and at ease with a partner. It speaks of an unconditional infant-type acceptance; of others completely accepting who we are, and vice versa, minus any invalidating critiques or judgements.

The Six of Cups can also indicate a re-emergence of emotionally charged people, places and events from the past, either in our thoughts or in physical reality. There in an indication of looking back at the past (Moon) in order to move forward with new, original or youthful ideas (Aces).

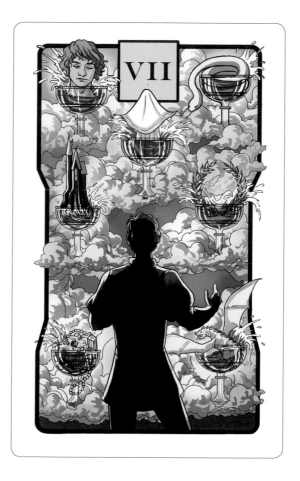

Seven of Cups

The Seven of Cups can indicate a scattered, unfocused or un-realistic approach to life, love, family, work, finances, health and well-being, being seduced by an illusion, born of many new ideas, energies and possible new identities (Aces).

However, in certain areas of business, the pursuit or creation of an illusion (Moon) or the possibilities that arise from an extra-fertile imagination can be practically applied (KP, QP) to win the day by mystifying the competition, using the element of surprise.

The Seven of Cups can also prove invaluable in the suspension of disbelief in an audience, which is key to the success of all fiction-based entertainment. However, on a personal level, our subjective truth should be tempered and balanced against objective reality to protect us from any fantastical fear-based ego-narratives (Devil).

Conversely, as a higher faculty of cognition, a clear and fertile imagination (KS, QS) is clearly distinguished from a subjective projection, reverie or fantasy (KnC, PC). It makes it possible for us to become aware of unseen spiritual forces in nature (High Priestess, 1C) and report back with great depth of clarity (Sun). This is a mystically minded card, concerned with all possible spiritual experiences related to the supreme, animating 'God' principle or creative force behind all faith religions, magic and mysticism.

A note of caution

The Seven of Cups in a relationship or any other type of reading can indicate a strong-felt but highly speculative, unrealistic, socially unfounded or groundless infatuation, fantasy or projection; essentially a mentally conjured romantic mirage. As such, this is not a good time to use the tarot or any other type of divination tool to convince yourself that any speculative situation or relationship is real, fated or destined.

Honestly distinguishing what is factually real from any wishful or delusory projections will ensure the preservation and protection of your socio-psychic integrity.

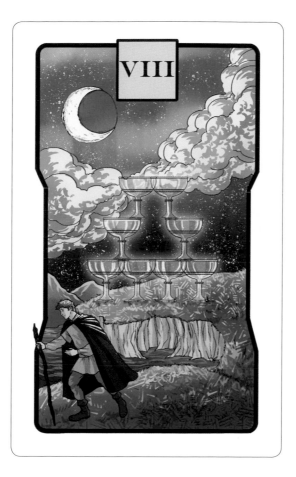

Eight of Cups

This is a card of seeking elsewhere, when what you want is yet to be found, or you are unclear to where, what or whom you, or your personal project, belong. The path ahead is unclear and unmarked, yet you refuse to let the obscurity deter you from your search.

In the darkness of night, nature's allotted time for growth, change and transformation, you may be questioning the validity of a previous path you chose to take. Ultimately, this questioning activates and initiates a new forward movement, which can only broaden your options, as it does your horizons. This is a journey worth taking, especially if, in some way, you are feeling physically, emotionally, socially or culturally underexposed. As the Eight of Cups is a card indicating underexposure in all its possible forms, it's likely you are looking for somewhere or some way to be yourself and truly shine. Your talents and abilities may have yet to find that right platform, support or encouragement. The people you would like to listen may be remaining inattentive or unsympathetic to your position, perspective or ideas.

But with every night there comes a dawn, and there is a sense with this card of knowing what you want and actively pursuing it, even if that means choosing to walk away from things you previously invested a great deal of time and energy in.

The Eight of Cups can also indicate that something fundamental to your health, happiness and contentment is missing. You could decide to walk away from a relationship or work situation that isn't working for you or, conversely, a partner or employer could turn away from you.

More often, though, this card appears when you are feeling energized, invigorated, strengthened and empowered by choosing to walk away from a situation that makes you feel hidden, weak, unfulfilled or lacking. Whether the decision is made by yourself or another, know it is beautifully orchestrated to set in motion your life's divine plan and purpose.

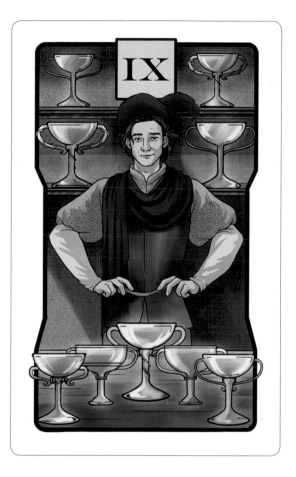

Nine of Cups

The Nine of Cups indicates a great feeling of success, prosperity, abundance, security, joy, happiness, contentment, satisfaction, well-being and adequacy in life, love, work, wealth, spirituality and health.

This card signifies the realizing of a dream, or deep emotional longing, which instils a real sense of meaning and purpose.

Whatever brings you the greatest emotional comfort, fulfilment and satisfaction is about to manifest, if it hasn't already. This is a time for reaping and enjoying the rewards of your previous effort and hard work. Something you sincerely wanted has come to pass. It is as if a magic wand has been waved over your life, fixing any issues or problems and lifting your spirits sky high.

The Nine of Cups indicates a great work, and doing what you are doing sets you apart from the rest. This is a time of achievement, reward and well-earned recognition. You meet your ambitions, reach a life goal, fulfil a cherished dream, wish or desire.

The Nine of Cups can signify a big promotion to a far more visible (Sun) or senior role (Emperor, Empress), or your thoughts, ideas, words (KS, QS), feelings, emotions (KC, QC), or material products (KP, QP) being very well received by another person, or the world at large (World).

In the position of the crossing card, or conjunct an unhealthy influence (Devil), your need for pleasure, satisfaction or gratification may be imbalanced, unhealthy and, ultimately, holding you back. As a card of self-gratification, the pleasing, satisfying, gratifying, entertaining, obliging or indulging of your moods, impulses, needs or desires may leave little room for self-discipline.

However, when surrounded by positively toned cards, the Nine of Cups indicates an emotional maturation period, where your personal strength, courage and power are increased via outgrowing your previous emotional support crutches.

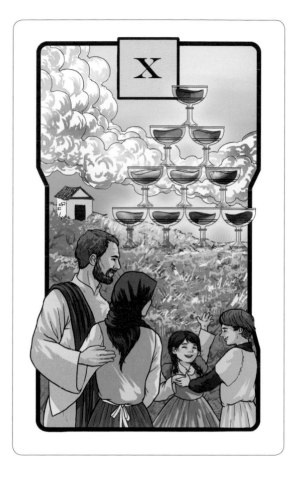

Ten of Cups

The Ten of Cups is indicative of the joy, happiness, peace, harmony, tranquillity, fulfilment and contentment that come from realizing your greatest hopes, goals, dreams, wishes and aspirations. It is a peak emotional experience, of a self-realizing nature, which leaves you feeling stronger, calmer, more peaceful and at ease than ever before. The success, prosperity and emotional security of this card are enhanced by feelings of meaning and purpose, or, in spiritual terms, a deep sense of divine alignment or at-one-ment with the universe.

When this card appears, it is likely that a deeply significant and perhaps long-held desire has been satiated. This can be the joy of starting or adding to a family, a declaration of true love, a marriage or a proposal, or simply the deep emotional fulfilment of an intimate relationship. Your intimate one-to-one relationships (2C) or business partnerships (2W) have progressed towards the final stage of completion by expanding and opening up to include your wider circle of loved ones or those who admire and covet your work.

Your goodness, optimism, inner light and beauty radiate outwards to positively impact and touch the lives of others. Gratitude for your blessings, whether in love, family, work, wealth or health, prompts a generous donation of your time and energy to others in your close-knit or wider community. As such, your interactions with friends, family, neighbours, co-workers and superiors are appreciative, supportive, friendly and satisfying, with all taking delight in your good fortune.

This is a card of completion and wholeness, of truly loving and embracing what life has given you. It is a card of being in the right place and the right space, mentally, emotionally, physically and materially, for your deepest desires to manifest.

Life works wonders when we are truly thankful and appreciative of its blessings.

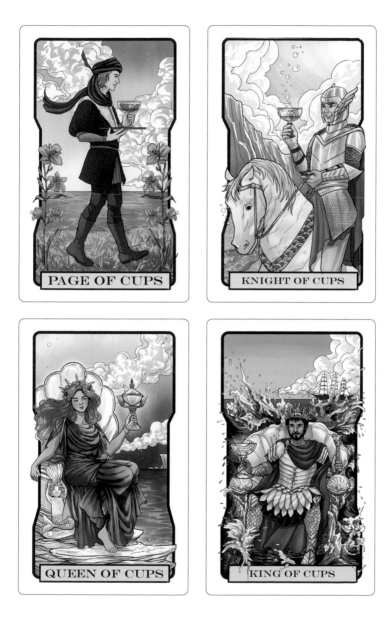

Cups Court Cards

The Cups courtiers are energetic representations of water energy at work in our life – or perhaps we are working it. All the court cards share the elemental motivations, agendas, desires and impulses pertaining to the ruling element of the suit to which they belong, but how each of the courtiers applies themselves to a situation depends on their individual level of development and maturity. The Cups courtiers are: the Page (PC), an immature or underdeveloped male or female energy or personality; the Knight (KnC), a moving-towards and outgoing male or female energy or personality; the Queen (QC) and King (KC), fully developed, realized, mature and established female and male energies or personalities.

The second plane of our alchemical human being is water, the immersive and absorptive element, represented by the suit of Cups, that transforms itself to perfectly fit any container, be it literal, like the human body, or personal, such as one personality, agenda or motive aligning with another.

In a similar vein to spiritual ambassadors or figureheads (High Priestess, Hierophant), the spiritually, empathically and compassionately motivated Cups courtiers are primarily concerned with relief of others' pain or the betterment of their life circumstances (6P).

The Queen of Cups, in particular, is a natural carer, adviser, counsellor and healer. The King and Queen's great emotional and spiritual maturity, grace, receptivity, endless patience, tolerance, unconditional love and accommodating attitude make them adept at drawing out the deepest hidden potential in others. Their kind words of encouragement are key when it comes to nurturing, nourishing and cultivating beginners or a project in the early stage of development.

The King and Queen are masters of conflict resolution, and their quiet diplomatic words can extinguish even the most blazing of arguments. Their social sensitivity, gentleness, empathy, collaboration, care and compassion for others make them valued, beloved and rewarding partners or leaders. Such is their ability to make others feel supported and protected, that they can do great work in fields concerning the mind, psychology or pathology. Their greatest personal satisfaction usually comes from social or welfare projects that directly address the needs of others. The Queen of Cups, in particular, develops unconditional compassion and unity consciousness by experiencing the world and everyone in it as a reflection of their own interior-state consciousness.

The Cups courtiers, like the element of water, are so adept at 'fitting in' that their own life, wants and needs are easily shaped and distorted by forces and energies that are more naturally assertive, moving and shaking (KW, QW), or unyielding (KP, QP). As water completely and utterly fits any vessel, container or space it enters, so the Cups courtiers seek to please by moulding and shaping themselves exactly to fit everyone and everything in their surroundings.

This amenable and accommodating nature is what makes it possible for these courtiers to show such great empathy, compassion, cooperation, compromise and consideration for others. However, they must guard against being too fluid, flexible, accommodating and obliging for the sake of peace-keeping and protecting others' feelings, for speaking their truth serves them better in the long run. However, those who specialize in increased palatability can make great cooks or chefs.

The Knight of Cups, in particular, is a passionate and eager romantic, tender, charming and forward with their emotions, but prone to forceful or intense idealism. In fact, both the Knight and Page's idealistic fantasies can soar way beyond what is usual in a relationship, to the point where they can feel deeply let down or disillusioned when a partner doesn't meet their ungrounded notion of how romantic relationships should be and feel.

The Page of Cups can indicate a playful, spontaneous, imaginative and joyfully childlike new relationship, or even the birth of a sensitive or emotional child. If difficult or challenging cards are present, this Page can indicate an emotionally immature or needy child or childlike individual who requires cyclical reassurance (Moon), nurturing, mothering (Empress) or constant care.

The King and Queen of Cups prefer to keep their deeper feelings to themselves, or the facts of a matter hidden, rather than be the bearer of a difficult or challenging truth. Just as water always takes the path of least resistance, its flow being directed by the lie of the land, the Cups courtiers, and the Knight of Cups in particular, work out how they are going to win someone over by continual mutual agreement, to the point of being overly obliging to them. This can make for a peaceful existence, albeit one where the Cups courtiers allow someone else's wants, dreams and wishes to shape and determine the flow of their life.

One of the greatest challenges for these courtiers is in fact losing the lineaments of themselves against others. Due to their liquid, mutable, metamorphic and absorbent personal boundaries, which enable the temporary hosting of another person's energy, they make brilliantly effusive or emotionally deep actors and performers. However, by providing a perfectly reflective surface upon which they mirror their surrounding environment, they may find their true selves, personal preferences and deeper desires remaining unfulfilled.

The Cups courtiers usually signify materially low-maintenance relationships that are reliant on a deep emotional or spiritual connection (2C) rather than the size of someone's wallet (KP, QP), public status (KW, QW) or intellect (KS, QS). Due to their inherent underrating of materiality, they remain true to their partner if and when their material or physical existence becomes tough. Therefore these courtiers can still thrive in circumstances in which those whose self-esteem is more status-oriented (KW, QW) or reliant on material satisfaction (KP, QP) would endure great suffering.

However, by relying on their surroundings for its own shape and form, the Cups courtiers need to watch for forming co-dependent relationships, where they allow someone else's psycho-emotional narrative, agenda and motivations to mould and shape their own. In romantic partnerships, Cups courtiers under negative influences (Devil) can take on the role of emotional or sexual feeders.

The priests of ancient Egypt never ate fish, or any other creature living completely immersed in water, which to them signalled a life lived hidden, or half-conscious. But fish move in mysteriously synchronized shoals and seem not to rely much on the world external to themselves for guidance; they have their own internal guidance system, and so it is with Cups courtiers. Where more intellectual (KS, QS, KnS), rational (KW, QW, KnW) or material (KP, QP, KnP) courtiers might see the information the Cups courtiers source as unreliable, there is a subjective, mysterious, unseen, unfathomable purity and depth to it, just as in the water-borne information found in our blood or DNA, or the new life present in liquid semen or an ovum.

The Cups courtiers are party to the great unknown secrets of the deep and are adepts at removing themselves completely to see the divine truth of a situation. They trust in higher guiding, mysterious or largely unknown sources, such as the wisdom of dreams, out-of-body exploration and extra-sensory perception. Placing their hope and faith in the inexplicable, unknown or unproven, and not being held back by the three-dimensional material world of facts, they allow themselves to be guided by their keen intuition and instincts. In fact, these courtiers can study and master all forms of spirituality and mysteries of the unconscious. They feel their way through life and are a barometer for personal, subjective or emotional truth, especially when the cognitive mind is in conflict with the heart, the driving force of the body's liquid-blood pumping system.

The Cups courtiers are the agents of a person's emotional or psychological state (Moon). The position these cards take in a reading shows whether our emotions are flowing freely, confidently and easily (1C, 9C, 10C), or dammed or sluice-gated to reduce their full force to a trickle, diverted below ground or via a longer, convoluted route, or simply stagnating in a pool (8S). As such, these cards are indicative of how directly or indirectly our feelings are expressed. If indirectly, they could be mistaken by a partner, or prospective partner, as apathy, impartiality or indifference (4C). But the personal life of the Cups courtiers is usually kept private; they are adepts at hiding their emotional attachments (2S), which can remain unacted upon for years, unless surrounding cards suggest the time is ripe for them to be revealed (Sun, 1C).

These courtiers often keep to themselves to themselves, living a somewhat secret, discreet or secluded life. Unless combined with high-visibility cards (Hierophant, Sun, World, KW, QW), they will happily remain under the radar, unseen, unheard or unnoticed (Moon, KC, QC). Such is the private nature of their own psyche that they often feel most comfortable in wild, remote, deserted, unfrequented sea or waterside locations; islands, retreats, sanctuaries, private homes, bathrooms and bedrooms. In fact they are highly sensitive, even over-sensitive (Moon), and may need to implement regular 'closing off' or 'down time' strategies to avoid being overloaded (10W) and burnt out (10S) by the busy, frenetic energies of the modern world.

THE SUIT OF PENTACLES

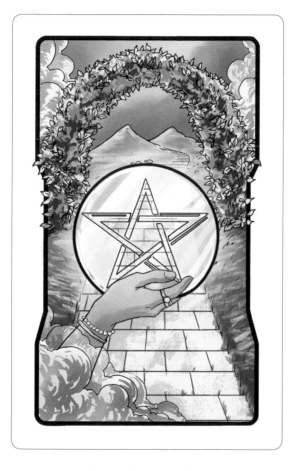

Ace of Pentacles

The Ace of Pentacles is indicative of a new financially or materially motivated beginning. It signifies that a new venture of some kind will bring greater levels of abundance and material gains further down the road. Your foundational plans are solidly laid and bound for success, due to your sensible, realistic, hard-headed, pragmatic, practical, no-nonsense, down-to-earth approach to life, love, business and health.

If you are upgrading, overhauling or relaunching a home, project, business or even relationship, this card is a strong indication that whatever time, energy or resources you invest now will be repaid with interest. When this card appears in a love, work or money reading, you have most likely backed the right 'horse'. This is a card of being right on the money, where you cash in on something you have supported, promoted, built, created or invested in. One successful opportunity begets other successful opportunities, as new business, revenue or resources come your way.

The Ace of Pentacles signifies that this is the optimal time for embarking on some new creative or financial speculation, and that the risk will pay off and put you in a position of greater strength. Any marketed property, or pitched projects or ideas, will be well received and/or sell quickly, and perhaps even for more than you expected to make.

The accrued value signified in this card doesn't have to be financial or material, however. It can be attributed to something you hold dear, such as a new, solid, socially grounded and stabilized relationship. It could be that a partnership, whether romantic (2C) or in business (2W), has brought greater all-round success and prosperity to your life.

In health matters, this card can indicate a pregnancy or the birth of a child. As Pentacles represent the physical body, this Ace indicates a fresh, new approach to your health and well-being, such as implementing a balanced exercise and nutritious dietary programme.

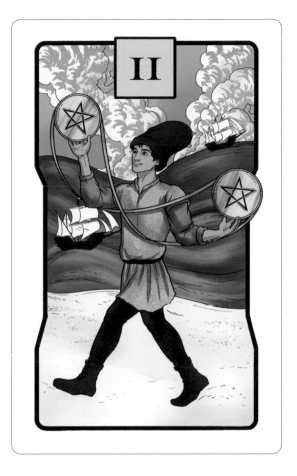

Two of Pentacles

The Two of Pentacles indicates finding balance, harmony and equilibrium during an unsteady or unsettled period of life, love, work, finances and health.

You may be juggling priorities, continually shifting your focus from one area of your life to another in an effort to keep your proverbial show on the road. There is a sense of riding the tides of change with this card, which can mean juggling work projects, resources or finances, or doing whatever it takes to keep your life on an even keel.

Remaining quick, flexible, adaptable, agile, attentive and focused are key to success and to the health of your mind, body, relationships and finances. However, you cope well with the swift or continual changes occurring in some areas of your life, and adopting a playful attitude gets you through even the worst personal or professional storms.

Spending quality time with a partner or your family may involve making a few adjustments to your work schedule or other social commitments. Conversely, you may be single because your many other commitments are holding you back from deepening a particular relationship. Spreading yourself too thinly can be an issue when this card appears, and is especially problematic in a relationship reading, as it indicates that your focus is on more than just one partner. As such, if cards of mistrust (7S) or underhandedness (Devil) are present, the Two of Pentacles can indicate double-dealing, cheating and extra-marital affairs.

In general, this is a card of playing it safe by hedging your bets. However, by remaining uncommitted or refusing to take a position on something, you will find your life will remain forever destabilized and unsettled. If you have been casually or hesitantly experimenting with different attitudes, positions, lifestyles, hobbies, creative modes, methods, disciplines, ideas, desires and speculations, it may be prudent to make a final choice, or find a balanced midpoint between them, if you wish to progress to the next stage by becoming established, recognized and rewarded in some area (3P).

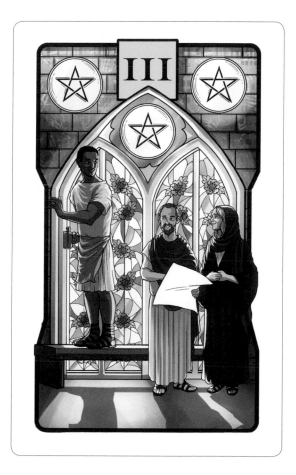

Three of Pentacles

The Three of Pentacles is a materially constructive card that indicates creating desirable things of lasting value, be they related to work, relationships, property or finance. Whether in a personal or professional reading, this card indicates that a mature, practical and cooperative attitude will help to create something beautiful and enduring. There is a sense of experienced people coming together for a shared cause or purpose, combining their perhaps diverse or varied skill sets and expertise to build, create or express something exceptional or uniquely different.

This is the card of personal or professional recognition, signifying a promotion, business contract, commercial transaction (Justice) or the powers that be approving your ideas and plans. It indicates being in a position to show the full range of your creative skills, talents, abilities, work or craftsmanship. There is an evolved and established artistry to whatever you apply yourself to at this time and the ability to elevate and turn even the simplest or crudest work into an art form.

This card suggests creative backing and inspiration, where sharing your biggest, wildest, most far-flung or long-term ideas, visions, aspirations and inspirations with an employer or benefactor brings professional success. There is a suggestion of finding, carving and crafting a distinct niche for yourself, or your product, in the wider world of commerce and business.

Others may have put their trust in you, or vice versa, with you delegating responsibility to your co-workers, with great results. The real-world, material or practical impact of your group effort is likely to be highly and widely regarded, and potentially have far-reaching influence (World, Sun).

On a spiritual level, this card gives a sense of using a conventional medium to express, or perhaps explain, the inexplicable, spiritual or ineffable, to give the natural forces of the universe that are seeking a form of material expression a pure, unadulterated birthing medium or channel.

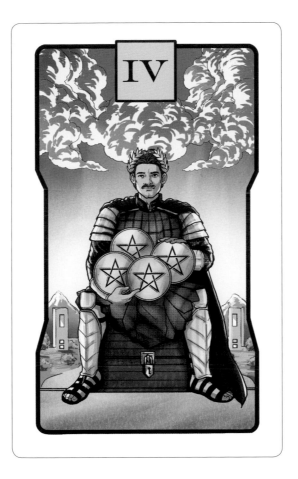

Four of Pentacles

The Four of Pentacles indicates someone renowned for living a moderate, unmaterialistic, no-frills life (Temperance) or being widely known as an austere, tight-fisted 'Scrooge' type who retains their sense of power and control (Devil, Emperor) by counting every penny.

This card indicates a situation where someone is being

extraordinarily frugal, conservative, cautious, careful or regulatory with their spending, finances and purchases, perhaps due to an innate, conditioned or imagined scarcity or poverty consciousness (Moon).

In a relationship reading, it indicates selfish or self-serving instincts with material resources and someone being ungenerous with spending, perhaps on themselves as well as others. As a result, when this card appears you may attract partners or relationships that create blocks or limitations around physical or material protection, home, shelter, nourishment, unconditional love and acceptance. Sadly, this card indicates a conservative form of generosity based on an estimate of your own or another's personal worth and value. It signifies the mistaken belief that our material wealth and acquisitions are the basis of our security and identity, hence why it is a card of coveting both possessions and people.

Fear of loss, whether it be of love, work, wealth or health, is likely to be proving a great obstacle to your progress at this time. By desperately clinging to the status quo, you may be making your life overly habitual and devoid of all spontaneity and originality.

One of the keys to happiness is the reduction and overcoming of the type of narrow-minded greed, suspicion and prejudice inspired by a deep fear of change. Greed, in particular, can create tremendous conflict in relationships.

Having a less entrenched and controlling relationship with the material world of resources, objects and people can help cultivate a nimble and unimpeded mind, with tremendous processing power (KS, QS, KnS).

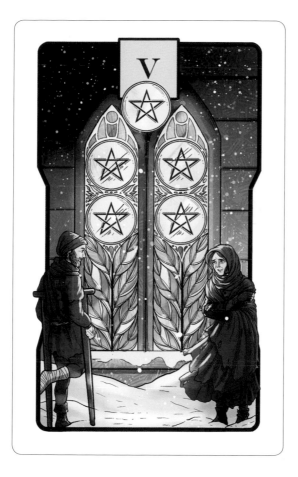

Five of Pentacles

The Five of Pentacles indicates a severe scarcity of money, resources or attributed value. Lack of acknowledgement of your worthiness makes relationships harder work than normal, and when this card appears, any recognition, credit or gratification due for your contribution to any endeavour will be demonstrably absent or feel impossible to earn.

There is an emotional coldness to this card, and you may be feeling the pressure of a significant social segregation or separation, either rejecting the company of others or being rejected by them. This card indicates being socially outcast, ostracized, excluded, shunned, ignored, snubbed, excommunicated, estranged, expelled, blackballed and blacklisted by a group or institution that, ironically, is itself becoming obsolete, having outlived its usefulness either to your own development or the evolution of the world at large.

If you are feeling isolated from particular friends and acquaintances, it is likely that you have spiritually outgrown them or their established norms, customs and practices. Though it can be hard, choosing to remain an outlier, operating on the outside and not as part of the majority, is a good test of the quality and strength of your integrity (High Priestess, KS, QS).

However, it is also possible that you yourself may be feeling left behind or forgotten and having to find your own way through without anyone else's help or assistance. You may be feeling alienated by your redundant employment status or the poor state of your material or financial affairs. This card indicates being turned down for loans or financial assistance.

However, it could also be that you have skills in scarce resource management (Emperor) or that a desperate lack of material resources inspires the implementation of a more efficient method of working, minus any waste or excess (1S).

The Five of Pentacles also signifies weakened immunity, vitamin deficiencies, depression (Moon, 9S), fatigue (4S), and physical aches, pains and injuries that could be partially remedied via a sojourn in a warmer climate.

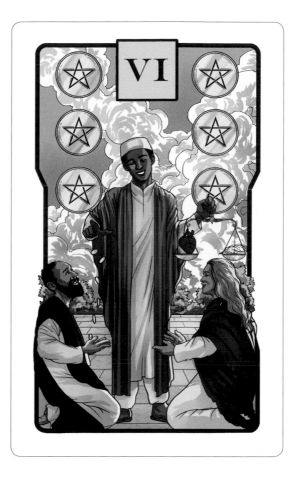

Six of Pentacles

The Six of Pentacles is a card of material success, profit and generosity of spirit. There is a sense of balance and equilibrium in this card, a balancing of extremely polarized positions when it comes to wealth, finances, and social standing or status. Whether you are the wealthy individual generously assisting others or they are assisting you, there is a sense of someone's position of power being used to better the life of another in need.

This card suggests that a noteworthy idea, project or proposition, which perhaps also has a useful, helpful, assisting, aiding, healing, curing, resolving or problem-solving incentive behind it, has been approved and backed by those with the power to make it happen. It indicates the pursuit of a noble, charitable or philanthropic cause, where those in positions of wealth and power are making decisions in accordance with their goodness and purity of heart, truth, order and justice.

The Six of Pentacles also symbolizes the success of all material or financial assistance applications, such as eligibility for a mortgage, business loan, social security, scholarships, awards, crowd funding, start-up backing, gifts and inheritances.

In a relationship reading, this card can indicate one partner supporting the other financially or materially, but, unless it is in the position of the crossing card, it is done in a spirit of caring, sharing and generosity. By resolving past issues and problems, this card instils a general all-round sense of comfort and security, where giving and receiving are done without any catch or expectation.

If you are single or dating, this card signifies encounters with generous-minded potential partners – those whose generosity extends beyond the sharing of their material resources.

Spiritually speaking, this card indicates a deep inclination to help and assist others in finding balance and equilibrium of mind, and purity of heart and purpose, through which the greatest possible healing can occur.

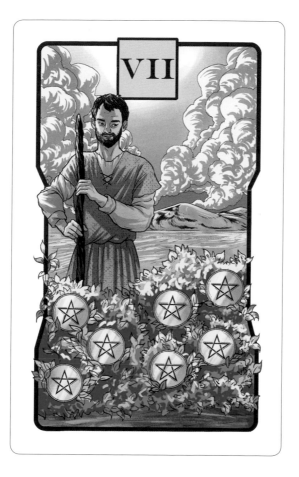

Seven of Pentacles

The Seven of Pentacles is a card of pausing to reflect, analyse, assess, appraise, review and evaluate your approach, efforts or performance in life, love, work, wealth or health. This is also time for hearing others' evaluations, learning from their and your own previous experience, and processing and taking stock of past failures and achievements.

This card suggests that success will come from standing back and allowing a person, relationship, creative project or product to grow, age, mature and evolve naturally, on its own, rather than from interfering. People, like plants, can't be forced to grow; they must be left to their own devices. This is nature's mandate. So, this mid-point card indicates a situation that requires much patience and perseverance before you can reap the greater rewards (9P, 10P).

The work you have done so far, be it on yourself or a material project, has borne fruit, albeit a modest harvest. Several options are available to you now and key practical decisions need to be made if your current endeavours are going to come to a fuller degree of fruition (10P). However, receiving this card well after a project or business transaction is complete indicates it is still capable of paying modest interest, royalties or dividends.

Practicality, pragmatism and applying what you have learned through direct physical experience are the keys to all future progress and expansion when this card appears, whether in love, work, wealth or health.

If you are single and looking for a relationship, this card provides an honest assessment of where you may have gone wrong in the past, and how you might better cultivate and nurture the love life you desire in the future. Partnerships, be they personal or professional, have most likely come a long way and proved somewhat satisfying when this card appears, yet there is still more work to be done.

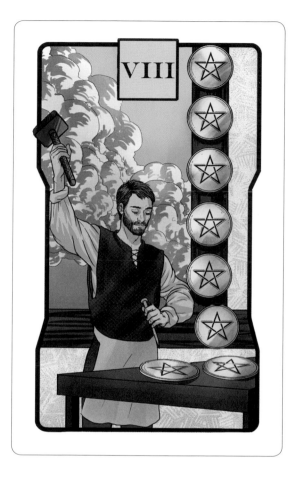

Eight of Pentacles

The Eight of Pentacles is a card of learning through direct experience and heeding life's lessons, whether these pertain to love, work, wealth or health. It signifies a period of instruction, study and training whereby old skills are honed, new ones acquired, and you learn by trial and error. This can apply to your own personal or spiritual education and development as much as a classroom, workshop, lecture, seminar or retreat-type setting.

The Eight of Pentacles is an enterprising and industrious card dedicated to the completion of a task or project, which may require a high level of production, manufacturing or engineering. This is a card of dedicated and diligent application, crafting, altering, improving and editing, as well as preparation, deliberation, order, precision, proficiency, efficiency, meticulousness, perfectionism, great observation, focus, concentration and attention to detail.

However, as a layout crossing card it can also indicate an unhealthy obsession (Devil) with alterations, order and perfection. Any physical, emotional, mental or general life imbalances experienced now may stem from having an obsessive single-point focus and unwavering determination to meet your own or another's high expectations.

When this card appears in a relationship reading, you and your partner are likely to be attentive towards each other, improving the relationship dynamic by learning how to better meet each other's needs. This will be a mutually instructive period, where you set about crafting your life together.

If you are single, this card suggests meeting someone in a studious or self-improvement setting or doing the necessary work on yourself to attract a satisfying relationship.

However, as a crossing card, the Eight of Pentacles can be too meticulous, exacting and detail-oriented. It may be you are passing up a potentially great offer, opportunity or relationship (4C) because it isn't the perfect fit or doesn't match your notion of the ideal scenario (7C).

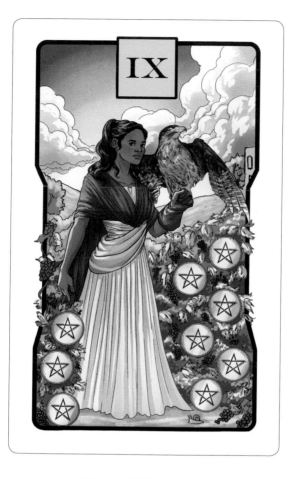

Nine of Pentacles

The Nine of Pentacles is the card of the accomplished self-made or self-employed individual, whose deep, unshakable core strength and resilience are cultivated via their self-sufficiency and self-reliance.

Wherever and however you have been investing your time and energy, the appearance of this card indicates that some sustained and persistent effort has or will prove more than worthwhile. Whether a creative or financial speculation has paid off or you have taken a major step up career-wise via a big promotion or other advancement, this card indicates the achievement of a higher position in life and all the material rewards that come with that. This is a card of upgrades, refinements, accomplishments, advances, elevations and a better quality of experience, be it in the personal, professional or any other sphere of life. There is a notable sense of the good life here, perhaps due to a wise use of your resources, combined with vision and foresight.

This card is likely to bring a significant increase in your material wealth, and signifies your enjoyment of elegant or refined sensual pleasures, material comforts and general abundance. If you have spent a great deal of time working towards a goal, the appearance of this card indicates that now is the time to enjoy the fruits of your labours. Such is your success in life, love, work, wealth and health that a more secure, solid and stable sense of your worth and value has been achieved.

Wealth and prosperity beget more of the same, and this card indicates the future success of a project, product or even relationship by projecting a solid sense of its worth and value.

On an interior or spiritual level, the beauty, peace, harmony, abundance and enjoyment depicted in this card indicate that you no longer rely on the opinions of others for your sense of self-worth. You can now turn your attention to higher-sourced forms of knowledge, applying the high-flying intelligence of a falcon to practical, material and mundane matters.

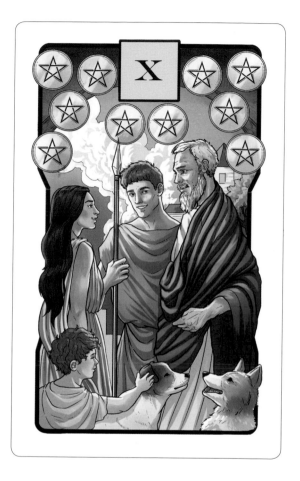

Ten of Pentacles

The Ten of Pentacles is a card of celebrating great worldly success, material wealth, abundance and prosperity, usually in the company of those you most value and appreciate. There is a great sense of material and family enjoyment, of security and belonging and freedom from financial restraints.

This card usually indicates large sums of money from business transactions, property and product sales, gifts or inheritances. The Ten of Pentacles can also signify great rewards, both of material or immaterial value, received for a long run of professional service, a long-standing relationship or marriage commitment, or any other remarkable feat of persistence and endurance.

Whether you are building or continuing a family legacy, there is a sense of continuation with this card, of a long-standing estate or business, treasured items, objects, ideas or values being passed on and preserved. However, the preservation of a family name and legacy may prove to be the proverbial gilded cage if this card appears in a crossing position, indicating the obstacle that is impeding your progress. In this position a desire for great wealth and the accompanying power and prestige may be blocking your path to true happiness and spiritual riches.

But under most circumstances, this card indicates the hugely successful completion of a major project or endeavour, both in material and immaterial/spiritual terms. Most people feel they have a material mission to fulfil in life, which is usually a task or problem to solve, the ramifications of which can positively affect many other people's lives as well as their own. In this sense, the Ten of Pentacles is a kind of humanitarian card, whereby great wealth has been amassed through ours or others' generosity to a cause or purpose that is beyond ourselves. The great success of this card is in the many lives its wealth touches and therefore improves, rather than just the few.

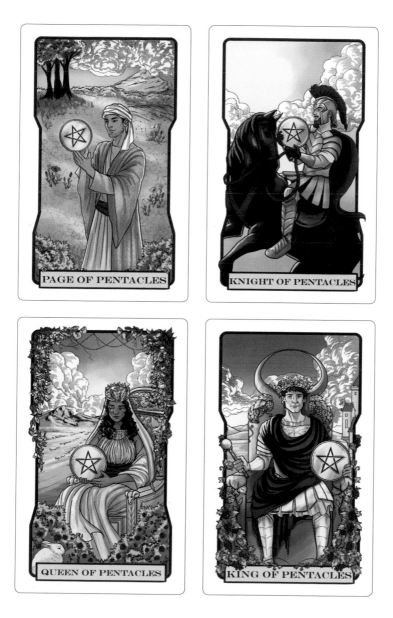

Pentacles Court Cards

The Pentacles courtiers are energetic representations of earth energy at work in our life – or perhaps we are working it. All the court cards share the elemental motivations, agendas, desires and impulses pertaining to the ruling element of the suit to which they belong, but how each of the courtiers applies themselves to a situation depends on their individual level of development and maturity. The Pentacles courtiers are: the Page (PP), an immature or underdeveloped male or female energy or personality; the Knight (KnP), a moving-towards and outgoing male or female energy or personality; the Queen (QP) and King (KP), fully developed, realized, mature and established female and male energies or personalities.

The third plane of our alchemical human being is earth, the solid, covering, constructive element of material matter represented by the suit of Pentacles, which, like the human body, is at once long-standing and recyclable.

In studying the qualities of earth, we get a sense of the permanent, reliable, enduring, practical, pragmatic ideology of the Pentacles courtiers. They do not or cannot understand, or even conceive of anything that they cannot see, hear, feel, smell or taste. This makes them more concerned with the sensual, material world than the intangible spiritual world, although a spiritually influenced (Magician, High Priestess) Pentacles courtier can produce wonderful divine materializations in fine art and craft form (Empress).

The Pentacles courtiers' primary concern is for financial and material prosperity, acquisition, ownership, gathering, hoarding, collecting, the accumulating of physical resources, money, capital, investments, precious and prized objects, and conveyancing, wealth or asset management, lineage values, and valuable connections and relationships.

As the overseers of all, the King and Queen prioritize the preservation, conservation and protection of their 'kingdom', no matter how big or small, domestic or national, social or professional. The appearance of these courtiers in particular signifies that the investment of time, energy or resources into a longer-term project is beginning to pay off.

Alongside other Pentacles cards, these courtiers indicate the slow and steady amassing of wealth and abundance, which in the longer term leaves you wanting for nothing, with no financial struggles, cares or concerns. When flanked by cards supporting their material values (10P, 9P), the Pentacles courtiers signify a good and comfortable life, lived in pleasing, opulent or luxurious surroundings – though this is the archetype most easily ensnared and owned by their material trappings, living life in the proverbial gilded cage (9S).

However, these understated courtiers are not as flashy with their cash or attention-seeking with their purchases as the fire or Sunlit cards (Sun, KW, QW, KnW, PW). They might buy a showpiece item or home, but as grounded, reserved, restrained, modest, unpretentious and moderate characters, they won't necessarily make anyone aware of it. Unless high-visibility cards are present, the Pentacles courtiers, who tend not to display or exhibit their passions and emotions, are easily eclipsed by more energetic or attention-commanding personalities (KW, QW, KnW).

If more dynamic cards are not present, the Pentacles courtiers tend to play it safe. They are creatures of the usual, ordinary and commonplace, who tend not to deviate from their routine, path, habits or tried, tested and so trusted things, people or places. When the Knight, in particular, goes out in search of something or someone, they can easily take the same route every time, and often know and stick to obtaining exactly what they set out to find. This trait can be applied to this card's search for a romantic partner: they know, and have perhaps always known, exactly what they want, and never consider anyone who falls even slightly outside their search criteria.

This can be applied to all the Pentacles courtiers to a certain extent, as the element of earth indicates a solid rigidity of purpose, which, spiritually speaking, blocks the light of greater awareness. These courtiers' sometimes heavy and serious nature indicates their tendency to be weighed down or physically anchored by negative, fear-based emotions. When these cards appear in a health-related reading, they indicate a time to relinquish material pressures, whether these relate to your own physical body and the need to lose weight, or releasing the tendency to allow wealth and materiality to dictate your happiness.

As practical and pragmatic rationalists, whose minds are anchored in mundane or material matters, the Pentacles courtiers often have superb and ultra-reliable organizational and problem-solving abilities. The King and Queen of Pentacles, in particular, indicate businessmen and women with an innate understanding of material reality and logistics and whose primary concerns expand profit margins (1P, 9P, 10P). If these cards appear in a work or business reading, it is likely that someone has identified a lucrative opportunity and is taking full advantage of it.

If you are looking for a financial backer for your project or product and either the King or Queen of Pentacles appears, it suggests someone is willing to take a calculated risk on you, and once they get involved, you can depend on them completely, for their word in business relationships, as well as personal ones, is as imperishable as the golden Pentacle.

When regulated and shaped by the Pentacles courtiers, the life-force energy flowing through us all is expressed in a way that seeks to build, reinforce or adhere to natural, earthly, practical and material laws, rules, structures and systems. The Knight of Pentacles, in particular, signifies all kinds of constructive critics, editors, craftsmen, precision technicians and engineers.

The Pentacles courtiers in general are constantly striving to improve and elevate the quality and value of something, be it a relationship, project or product. The Page of Pentacles indicates the taking of practical and realistic initial steps, either via studious or scholarly research, which will offer material rewards further down the road. The Queen of Pentacles warmly and generously, but also practically, mothers, nurtures and nourishes people and projects in order to bring out, develop and build on their attributes and qualities. The steadfast, home-loving and practical Queen provides stable shelter, comfort and nourishment for all who need it.

Thought these courtiers are generally not as communicative as the Wands or Swords suits, the Page of Pentacles still represents messengers, emails, letters, texts and all forms of communications bringing news on physical or material matters.

The King of Pentacles tends to speak in indirect and practical, rather than emotional (Cups), passionate (Wands) or logical (Swords), terms about their feelings. However, not verbally expressing their feelings, or actively pursuing a prospective partner, should not be taken as impartiality or indifference, unless otherwise indicated (4C). On the contrary, the depth and sincerity of the King's, Queen's and Knight's feelings are not fathomed by words or conversation (Swords), a show of emotion or feeling (Cups) or great displays of affection (Wands), but more by the practical perfection of the dates or outings they plan and the money, resources and time they invest in a relationship.

They want their partner to share in their love of the best-quality sensual experiences, whether these involve eating and drinking or enjoying luxurious surroundings. The Pentacles courtiers' relationship agenda is often to find a life partner who, like them, most values the quality and perfect order of an experience, as well as the practical accumulations of wealth and property.

No matter what the situation, the Pentacles courtiers are greatly respectful, responsible, steadfast and trustworthy. Whether they appear in a relationship, work, wealth or health reading, these courtiers can be relied upon to show prudence, care, caution, hesitation, calculation, pragmatism and practicality. If you are primarily seeking a great practically minded, provider-type partner, these courtiers will not disappoint you.

THE SUIT OF SWORDS

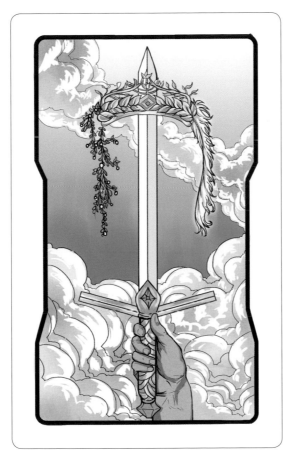

Ace of Swords

The Ace of Swords can indicate conceptual intellectual empowerment, such as coherent and intelligent verbal articulations or literary expressions. It is the invocation of force that drives us to courageously speak out or verbally fight for an original thought, cutting-edge idea or greater cause. It is the sharp clarity of thought, awareness or genius (Sun) behind innovative, original, inventive, universal (World) or inspired processes (Star).

Also known as the Sword of Truth and Discernment, the Ace of Swords cuts through the veils of illusion held in place by the fearful shadow aspect of the mind. Cutting through the superficial overlay of our ego personality, it uncovers our core identity.

In the intellectual pursuit of truth and justice, this Ace assures victory. It solves problems and overcomes challenges by quickly and keenly cutting to the chase. The new ideas or information it uncovers brings far greater clarity of heart, mind and purpose.

The Sword is swift and merciless in cutting any painful ties that bind us to the past. Though ruthless, this necessary severance with the past is what enables a new chapter of life to begin. Being forced to start again, to rebuild, perhaps from scratch, may bring far greater and more efficient results. What enables us to move courageously forward and begin again after a struggle is the ability to sacrifice that which no longer serves our highest good and greater purpose.

The Ace of Swords is ultimately a healing agent in its cutting, severing and detaching, distancing us from our old limitations and blockages. It is especially useful in instigating the change needed to heal and/or modernize any outdated work, health or relationship arrangements. However, as the proverbial double-edged sword, it can cut both ways, and often bestows its favourable results via some difficulty and challenge.

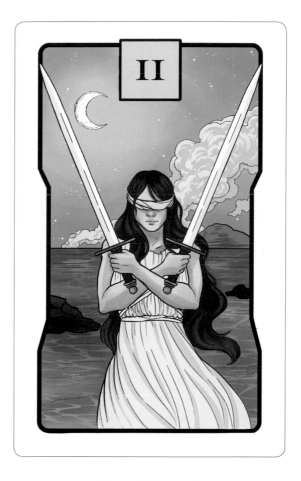

Two of Swords

The Two of Swords represents the discomfort that comes from an internal or external clash of ideas; where two parties, in either a romantic or business partnership, are refusing to compromise. When this card appears, you might find your unique self-expression – the path of the heart – is being blocked or clashes head on with the path of another. The Two of Swords indicates a situation where agreeing to disagree is the only option to keep the peace. Whether the conflict is internal or external, by not compromising your vision just to indulge or oblige those who may have a different outlook or opinion, you keep your integrity strong and intact.

The heart centre, being protectively crossed, signifies that you are already holding your ground and guarding your truest and highest interests. This can include not adhering to a particular lifestyle; not following the crowd or a cultural fashion trend; adhering to a particular point of view or school of thought; not taking sides, using clichés or following stereotypes; and not sticking to a particular types of friends, associates or romantic partners.

As one of the 'blinkered' cards, the Two of Swords suggests living in ignorance or turning a blind eye to certain matters that are calling for your attention. You are likely to be at a cross-roads, stuck in a period of stasis or impeded by a stalemate situation. This card marks ambivalence or indecision, not know-ing which way to go (Moon). The decision regarding a relationship, business, financial or health matter may not be taken (or agreed) for some time yet (Hanged Man).

Sometimes the more diplomatic and tactfully intelligent approach (Strength) is to entirely disengage from any conflict or fractious situation by staying wholly self-contained. Whether this indicates real inner strength (Strength) or cowardice and fearful aversion (7S, 8S, 9S) depends on the surrounding cards.

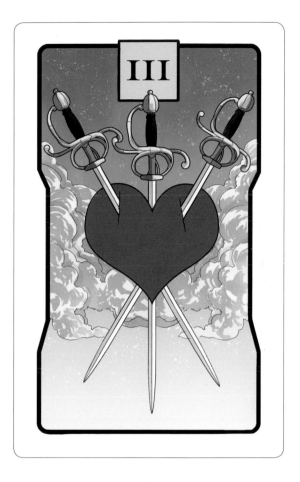

Three of Swords

The heart, in the centre of the body, radiates our core truth, and we can only feel truly alive by speaking our heart's truth. If we are disregarding our heart's intelligence by being untrue to our core desires, it must work harder to make itself heard. Whether emotional or physical, this is what causes our greatest heart-ache, and heartbreak.

291

Only an untrue heart can be seriously hurt by the truth, and yet the truth then becomes a creatively-destructively principled force. This is the numerological nature of the Three of Swords. Its higher purpose is to help enlighten a heavy heart burdened by the mind's untruths.

When our consciousness is heavy as a result of not facing the truth of a situation, the heart will seek to protect itself from any force that opposes its morally honest and incorruptible qualities. The Three of Swords indicates that impurely reached decisions, and motivations and agendas born of our clouded head rather than heart centre, are being dissected and cut out by the three creative Swords of Truth.

The critical point behind this card is to help us determine whether our actions, thoughts, motivations, agendas and even identity are appropriately balanced and centred with our innately higher-minded heart. Heart-centred actions are pure, straightforward and devoid of any mental or intellectual convolutions.

The tarot's transparency can sometimes be cutting, but by heeding these lessons, we can make our life's journey one of greater integration and cooperation, rather than a painful meeting of the mind and heart. Greater truth is always to be found within the heart; whether it is welcomed and accepted, seated and centred, or unwelcomed, unaccepted and painfully placed there by force is up to us.

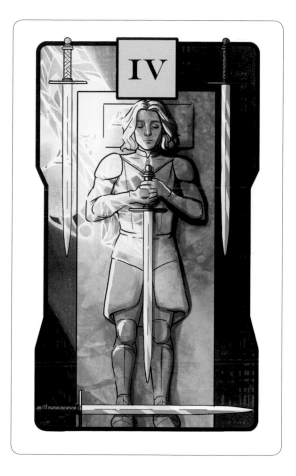

Four of Swords

The Four of Swords indicates a time of peace, calm, tranquillity and intellectual repose found within yourself rather than in external sources. When this card appears, by finding a private space in which to withdraw, you will find this self-improving act of ritual isolation provides the much-needed time out when you can think, contemplate, meditate,

293

recharge, replenish and rehabilitate your health and strength of purpose.

When morale is low or you are feeling a bit flat, quiet time away from it all, perhaps on a secluded holiday or in a sanctuary or retreat, boosts your energy and improves your general mood and outlook. However, it is wise to put a time limit on this, as going too far into yourself and becoming a victim of your own self-absorption can deepen depression.

Conversely, isolating yourself from those who are a damaging, negative or harmful influence, and who perhaps overindulge in harmful activities, will make your recovery all the quicker. As a card of withdrawal, the Four of Swords does include the symptoms experienced when the effects of addictive substances, activities and even people begin to leave our system.

There is also a suggestion of going into hiding, perhaps through shame or embarrassment. Preferring to keep your own counsel and not allowing your problems to become anyone else's are key attributes of growing, ageing and maturing pains.

It may be that you need to take a break from a close relationship, to mentally or emotionally withdraw from someone to overcome deep wounding or emotional exhaustion. Fortunately, this card indicates a tough and lonely time becoming gradually easier, especially after the complete cutting of ties (1S) with any old, outdated or obsolete sources of care, love and affection (Moon, 5C, 3S).

The Four of Swords may also suggest a withdrawal from the material world to find spiritual guidance. It indicates that taking care of your own spiritual needs and wants should come first and foremost at this time.

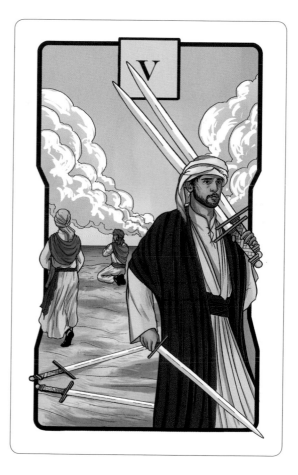

Five of Swords

The Five of Swords is the card of winning the battle, but not the war. This card indicates a degrading, dishonest and self-defeating victory or a hollow rejoicing in others' misfortunes that sets us up for losing out overall.

All negative thoughts have a psychic weight, so psychically storing up and carrying others' offences, perhaps with a plan to redress them at a later date, only impedes our spiritual and life progress. Even self-defeating motivations, such as trying to impress others by doing the 'right' or noble thing, can backfire, because our ego attachments are then a by-product of our morally correct behaviour. Yet being too forceful, aggressive, competitive or desperate to win, no matter what the cost (Chariot, 6W), only leads more directly to pain and suffering.

The Five of Swords generally indicates a separation from others, perhaps due to an overly harsh critique. Disarming others with cold or harsh but nonetheless true words may have left you alone. You may have won the battle, but alienated others in the process.

Conversely, agreeing with others and taking on their ideas to avoid open conflict or settle an argument compromises your overall psychic integrity.

Sometimes we do and say anything to avoid being the bearer of bad or unpleasant news, though this only keeps ourselves and others in a kind of temporary unconscious comfort zone (Moon).

This card indicates the trap of winning a fight by promoting or backing the questionable words and actions of others: an approach that serves no one in the long term. True love and respect contain the ideology of a truthful commitment and having the integrity to selflessly serve someone's best interests (High Priestess), however unpleasant or uncomfortable that may be.

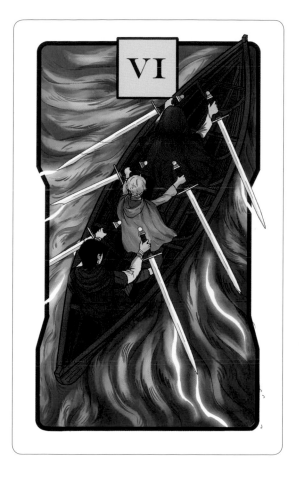

Six of Swords

When the Six of Swords is present in a reading, a new-found stability of thought cuts through our old turbulent emotions to keep us buoyant, balanced and moving forward. It could be considered a rite of passage that marks some form of literal or figurative transition in our life.

This card indicates that others' challenging yet constructive criticisms have been integrated and taken on board, and helped us to improve our life and prospects. When there are problems that need solving, whether they be personal or professional, the Six of Swords steers us towards calmer emotional waters, where we can progress more directly to a solution.

The Six of Swords also indicates a need for new places, faces and life experience. Though the journey may be slow, or taken in incremental stages, it will succeed in putting distance between us and any past difficulties.

It could be that you are poised to take an entirely different course in life, a course that may involve overseas travel (KnW), international projects or foreign affairs. This card indicates the paradigm shifts that result from journeying to new worlds, and so represents all scientific, exploratory or experimental undertakings. Some adventure into new territories of experience, either literal or figurative, is being undertaken now – an adventure that knows no bounds or is inspired by the unknown. As such, this card indicates using a balance of intelligence and intuition to ensure progress.

The Six of Swords also brings forth the future via far-flung ideas, perhaps ones that others have yet to conceive of or appreciate. Whether these ideas have merit, are found credible by others and so implemented successfully in a relationship, work project or society depends on the outcome cards: the outcome of the journey.

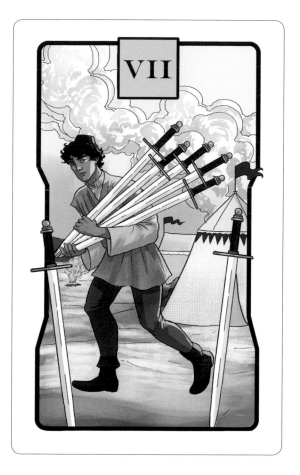

Seven of Swords

In the Seven of Swords a lone man walking away from his camp, carrying more than just his own sword, suggests there is a situation in your life that is born of, or requires, a surreptitious, shady, dishonest, covert, hidden, undercover, clandestine, stealthy or veiled approach.

Everything in the tarot is an aspect of ourselves. The people lying unaware in the tents are the unconscious aspects, while the unexposed figure carrying other people's ideas and thoughts (Swords) is a semi-conscious aspect. When we look at our own feelings and beliefs about ourselves, how many of them can we say are truly our own and not unconsciously adopted, absorbed or taken verbatim from those who are projecting their own internal issues onto us?

With the appearance of this card, behind the scenes actions can also be happening in your semi-conscious or unconscious mind. The card's presence reminds you to look at your own beliefs about yourself and work out what is true and authentic, and what you have unconsciously picked up from others. When a man is depicted as carrying others' swords, he is really carrying their thoughts, concepts and ideas about himself, and allowing them to co-create his own self-concept.

By unconsciously carrying around the negatively weighted thoughts of others, which don't innately belong to you, you will find your spiritual or life progress impeded. Shedding this overly weighted self-concept will allow you to see who you really are beneath your conditioning. This is the definition of en-lightenment healing.

This card indicates it's time to en-lighten the load on your mind (10W) by discarding any second-, third-, fourth-, even fifth-hand beliefs about yourself and others. Wherever these have come from – parents, family members, friends, school-teachers or whoever – it's time to recognize what extraneous information no longer serves you and discard it.

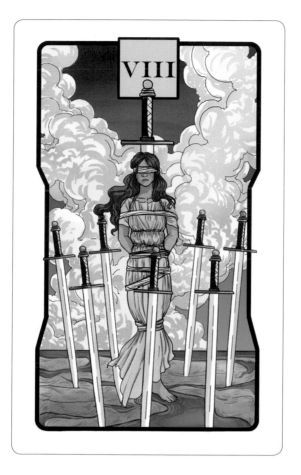

Eight of Swords

The Eight of Swords can indicate debilitating health challenges caused or exacerbated by a refusal to acknowledge them, or ignoring the unhealthy aspects of our life. It represents a feeling of immobilization due to an unconscious fear of love, abandonment, rejection or conflict. It is a self-inflicted period of stagnation that comes from self-limiting doubts, beliefs and expectations, rigid fear of change or fear of making a wrong decision.

In order to free ourselves from the psychological ties that blinker and bind, the Eight of Swords draws our attention to those unconsciously inhibiting aspects of the self, the aspects that render the otherwise progressive psyche paralysed by its own unnecessary fears and anxieties.

The Eight of Swords is comparable to finding our progress in life blocked by the psyche's obscuring ego forces, which are unable or unwilling to see the light of truth. The cage-like barrier of swords symbolizes the forces in our psyche that prevent us from becoming self-realized (Magician, High Priestess, Sun) or attuning to the higher truth of our situation.

If we allow it, however, the swords can act like clearing objects, freeing us from the cage of our mind by mercilessly cutting through the psychical dirt, grime and blockages. This card expresses the potential for such self-liberation, with the figure being tied to the Sword of Truth and Justice itself (1S).

The Eight of Swords prompts us to recognize that we all hold the means of our own escape, for it is our own blind, blinkered and self-sabotaging mindsets and thought processes that have entrapped us in the first place.

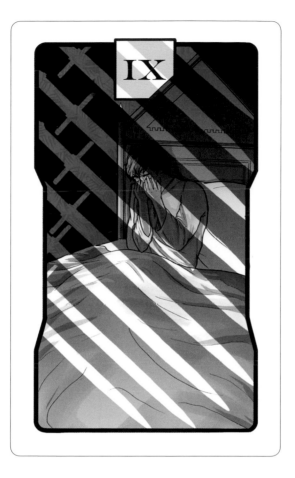

Nine of Swords

The Nine of Swords can indicate obsessive overthinking as a by-product of our physical inaction or idle intellectualism, or mental pessimism, expecting or imagining (Moon) the worst (Tower, Death), and the difficulties we face from having such a negative outlook.

It could be that an oversaturation of toxic anger, sadness,

bitterness, resentment, grief and guilt is keeping us emotionally self-imprisoned. Living in dread of what negative things may happen, afraid that any change in the status quo may make things worse, we can become ever-more withdrawn, nervous, anxious and divorced from the brighter side of life.

When our life-force energy dips and dims, our sublime conscious mind is obscured. In the darkness, we experience a loss of will-power, conscience and even heart. Emotional heartbreak, or a physical problem with the heart or the life-giving reproductive organs, can then be the result (3S).

When our mind becomes fixed on insatiable egocentric or materialistic endeavours, happiness, joy and optimism remain elusive. The ego, however, revels in the dramatization of pain and cerebral self-torture. We plague ourselves with doubt, fear, guilt and shame over our own and others' past wrongs, misdoings or catastrophic losses. Animosity, resentfulness or embittered feelings towards the past or a current situation keep us psychologically imbalanced, unrested or restless. We can thoroughly exhaust ourselves by continually reciting our own self-justifications in opposition to a broken business or relationship agreement. For the conscious individual – who can accept responsibility without any projection of blame – the pain of an injustice can be significantly reduced. Otherwise, we can waste much time indulging our own troubles and remain enslaved to our victim mentality for years.

By accepting and integrating the lessons of the Nine of Swords, we can avoid any future repetitions of such painful 'nervous breakdown' cycles (Moon, Tower).

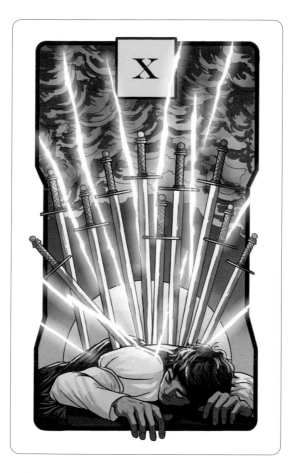

Ten of Swords

In the Ten of Swords, the desperate overthinking we saw in the previous card has resulted in a cerebral mind-crash, where our over-intellectualizing, yielding too much information and making too many connections, has gone beyond the point of sustainability.

When this card appears in a reading, the harsh critiques of

others about how a person or project appears can ultimately transform it for the better. Perhaps the critic or editor is you, hunting out and mercilessly correcting your own or others' perceived imperfections.

An unnecessary aspect of yourself, which is likely to have been causing you great internal and external trouble and strife, is now brutally attacked and killed off, allowing for a complete overhaul and refinement of your personality and character.

Acts and pursuits leading to the ruin or undoing of our ego often persist until the old self has been successfully released and that cerebral cycle has come to an end. Although for the conscious self-observer, the harshest critiques can enforce the swiftest and most efficient identity changes.

Human restlessness and the urge to cyclically re-enact our own self-destruction are what make us so psychologically complex as a species. Our self-destructive behaviour may manifest as the result of some form of initiation, spiritual or otherwise, with the intention of consciously relinquishing our outdated ego attachments.

Sometimes, psychological trauma can result from redefinitions of the self that have been forced upon us by external pressures or events. However, when the Ten of Swords is surrounded by positively toned cards, the transformation that ensues from any sudden changes in our core identity will ultimately be for the good of all concerned.

As vegetation grows, changes and transforms itself during the night, so we, as humans, suffer the growing pains of our own cerebral flowering in the darkest moments of our life.

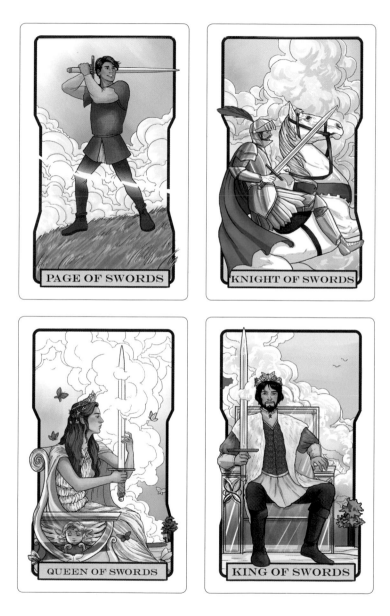

The Swords Court Cards

The Swords courtiers are energetic representations of air energy at work in our life – or perhaps we are working it. All the court cards share the elemental motivations, agendas, desires and impulses pertaining to the ruling element of the suit to which they belong, but how each of the courtiers applies themselves to a situation depends on their individual level of development and maturity. The Swords courtiers are: the Page (PS), an immature or underdeveloped male or female energy or personality; the Knight (KnS), a moving-towards and outgoing male or female energy or personality; the Queen (QS) and King (KS), fully developed, realized, mature and established female and male energies or personalities.

The fourth plane of our alchemical being is air, or the subtlety of gases. This is where our mind and soul transcend the physical bodily planes of earth and water to once again join with the subtlest element, air, represented in the tarot by the suit of Swords.

The Sword courtiers easily grasp subtle, symbolic, metaphorical, abstract or intangible concepts and have an acute perception and appreciation of dry humour and social, dramatic, literary or artistic subtexts. Compared with the other suits, who use physical actions (Wands), emotions (Cups) or resources (Pentacles), the Swords courtiers rely on logical or visual presentations to make an argument.

The keen logic, intuition, insight and perception of the Swords suit, and of the Queen of Swords in particular, can know no bounds; penetrating any deception or confusion and seeing straight to another's core concerns. However, in certain card pairings the Swords courtiers become classic overthinkers (10W, 8S, 9S): over-perfecting (8P), over-analysing (7P), finding subtexts, subtle suggestions, intimations, insinuations, hints or hidden agendas: seeing through everything (Fool, Moon, KnC, 7C).

In particular, the constant mental traffic of the Page of Swords, who is an eager conversational information-gather, can fuel chronic indecision (Moon, 7C) or prompt the premature enacting of embryonic ideas.

However, without any circuitous or convoluting emotional or material influences, the Sword courtiers' signature success lies in their swift, sharp and astute decision-making. When something, or someone's behaviour, begins to feel outdated, untruthful or unethical, the Knight in particular can swiftly move on, severing ties and not looking back. The Knight is also open, clear, frank and direct in their speech, always 'cutting to the chase' or getting quickly and efficiently to the point.

Being forward focused, the Swords courtiers' ideas are the original 'cutting-edge' concepts behind creative acts or expression (Sun), the energy source behind a fresh communicative messaging style, narrative, handcraft, way of writing, instruction or arrangement of information.

Their acuity and eloquence of speech is partly due to their ultra-connective and incisive intellect's ability to swiftly recall and synthesize information, but also the result of their clean mental processing.

The term 'incisive', meaning 'intelligently analytical and clear-thinking', comes from the same etymological source as 'incision', hence the reason for using a sword blade to symbolize the air element. Personified, the Knight of Swords in particular can be a fearlessly incisive editor, critic or commentator, whose views, unfettered by emotional (Cups) or material (Pentacles) concerns, are accurate and focused.

All these courtiers can be writers or artists (Empress), whose work offers incisive views or images of cultural events. Paired with the Wands, they can indicate quick, direct and unimpeded thoughts turning to incisive moves or actions (KW, QW, KnW).

The Sword courtiers live and die by the Sword of Truth, when their life philosophy of clarity and transparency at all costs gets them out of, but also into, trouble and strife. They symbolize our intellectual ability to recognize the true nature of things by giving names to them. However, on the whole, being true to themselves and defending (9W) or upholding truth, justice and transparency are key to retaining their own or others' sense of integrity, which brings them the greatest overall joy and happiness (Sun, 10C).

The King of Swords, in particular, is a calm, fair, forthright, incorruptible and indisputable judge, whose ethical approach, unfettered by emotional or material concerns, allows them to understand both sides of an argument, which in turn inspires absolute trust in their judgement.

The idea that a dry soul is the wisest of souls was first conceptualized by the ancient Egyptians. They called the divine air that pervades all of space and the wider universe, Maat, a word synonymous with 'truth' and 'order'. This is due to the air element's clarity and transparency, allowing the light of the Sun directly through it to illuminate, enlighten, animate and enliven the world around us. Without the air element, earth blocks the light of the Sun, and so does water, depending on its depth and degree of clarity distortion. This same principle applies to the human condition, as our earthly existence can dim or be distorted, or, when the air element is present, allow our pure, radiant, enlightened inner spirit to shine forth (Sun) like sunlight through a clean window pane.

The elder Swords courtiers, the Knight, Queen and King, have a clear and sharpened consciousness devoted to transparency and truth. The mandate of their incisive, cutting minds is to reveal what is hidden by piercing or slashing the veil of illusion that obscures the true reality. They fiercely detect, and set about dissecting and removing, any shadowy, distorting or obscuring elements in the psyche (Devil, Moon), fighting against the opponents of truth and visibility. This can often be a painful process, not just for themselves, but also for those close to them, those who are not used to looking at themselves so directly.

Due to their strong sense of integrity, the Swords courtiers can also be frank and outspoken, but always with great purity of purpose: to restore justice and set things to rights. The King and Queen are usually masterful diplomats, but the Knight and Page of Swords can sometimes be perceived as going too far and saying too much. However, if you are on the receiving end of a cutting truth, it is worth remembering that it takes a great deal of integrity, bravery and courage to put truth and justice above a personal need (Moon) to be liked or popular.

Yet in relationship questions, the Swords courtiers can indicate a period of emotional coldness, hard truths and the exposure of unsupportable assumptions and expectations within a relationship, which force those who are single or in a partnership with co-dependent tendencies to become more interdependent and self-reliant.

How the Swords courtiers' truthful perceptions are received depends on the self-awareness and general level of consciousness of the recipient. If the information is gracefully or tactfully delivered (Strength) or tempered to meet the level of compassion required to be effective (Temperance), the Swords courtiers can package useful personal development information in a way that greatly engages and appeals to others (Empress, Sun).

Their emotional aspect is often overruled by their powerful will and the intensity of their intellect, which can exact a great and powerful influence. However, they can reside too much in their head and not enough in their heart. Despite their incisive insights, they tend to lack the empathy necessary to be effective counsellors. They are more suited to medical, humanist or humanitarian causes, academia, writing, investigative journalism, law, order or justice systems, or any profession where they can honestly and directly enlighten, inform, create transparency or draw attention to the truth with their dissecting thoughts, words and views.

Fired by exacting perfectionism, the Knight of Swords, in particular, can have an exceptionally reactive counter-corrective tendency. So, when these cards appear, we may be on the receiving end of another's critically incisive or verbally cutting judgement – perhaps a final judgement (Judgement). If we have spent our life indulging aspects of ourselves that are untruthful, we are likely to experience the Sword courtier's words as painfully revealing.

Overall, however, what the Swords symbolize is the cutting back of the overgrown ego, and once these unconscious or wayward aspects have been exposed to the light of our conscious mind (Sun), the unconditional joy, happiness and contentment of our enlightenment and healing can commence.

TIME-EFFICIENT TAROT CARD LAYOUTS

As a professional tarot reader, I only ever use five layouts when doing readings for myself or a client, and I have included them all in this book. I have found these layouts to be the most useful for our modern-day interests, concerns and sensibilities. Some are traditional layouts, others more recently invented, yet all offer a unique perspective on the insights and answers sought by the reader.

Whether you are just beginning to read the cards or are already an experienced reader, you will find all these readings, bar the relationship reading, can be used to answer any question or provide insight into any area of your life.

A SINGLE CARD OF THE DAY

Refresh the page of your mind. Be an agent of the unthinkable. Beat algorithmic automation! To spice up life, try choosing a tarot guidance card and letting it shape your day, month or even year. Completely relinquish control and find true freedom by picking a card at random and letting that card decide your fate. The tarot can move and shake your life, or a specific area you are wishing to activate, and perhaps take you somewhere deeply surprising.

So, for students and experienced readers alike, it can be useful, upon waking up in the morning, to shuffle the deck, then blindly and randomly, with the picture side facing down, select a single card to provide a little foresight on the energies at work during the day ahead. This is an excellent way to learn more about each individual card, as when the day is coming to a close, you have the perfect opportunity to analyse the day's events and see how they were reflected in the card.

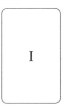

A word of caution
Don't fall into the self-fulfilling prophecy trap by selecting the morning card then going out of your way to make those events

happen. That doesn't serve anybody. Instead try to be a passive observer, while using the benefit of foresight to navigate the day's energies with greater conscious awareness.

THREE-CARD LAYOUT

This is a bit of a classic, and the most time-efficient layout if you are reading for a group or need to cover a lot of separate areas or questions in a short space of time. Following the instructions on how to read the cards at the beginning of the book (*page 13*), lay three cards in the positions below:

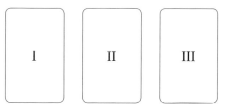

I. Past: the defining event or energy of the past that subsequently influenced and shaped present and future events
II. Present: what is happening right now, as a result of past influences, and what will happen in the future as a result, although sometimes efforts can be made to change the outcome
III. Near-future outcome: what will happen as a result of past and present actions, energies, events and influences

FIVE-CARD LAYOUT

Another time-efficient layout, but one that adds a depth to the reading, is the five-card layout. Following the instructions on how to read the cards at the beginning of the book (*page 13*), lay five cards in the positions below:

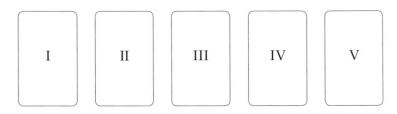

I.   Past: the defining event or energy of the past that subsequently influenced and shaped present and future events

II. Past: another significant influence that helped shape the present moment

III. Present: what is happening right now, as a result of past influences, and what will happen in the future as a result, although sometimes efforts can be made to change the outcome

IV. Hidden aspect: what hidden or unconscious forces are at work in the situation (or perhaps you are working them!)

V.   Near-future outcome: what will happen as a result of past and present actions, energies, events and influences

Future Extension Cards

If more information is required, extension cards can be added to this reading by spreading the remaining deck of cards, picture face down, across the table and randomly selecting a few more cards – between three and five more. These cards should be read as an extension of Card V (near-future outcome), except they represent the more distant future possibilities that will become apparent as time progresses.

TEN-CARD CELTIC CROSS LAYOUT

The ten-card layout adds even greater depth to the reading and specifically indicates what energies, events and influences are holding you back or impeding your progress. Following the instructions on how to read the cards at the beginning of the book (*page 13*), lay ten cards in the positions opposite:

I.   Present signification: the present driving and defining force, influence or event that is inspiring the reading

II. Crossing card: what positive or negative energy, influence, event, challenges, impedes, holds back or opposes you or your progress

III. The crown: obvious and conscious influences; the shaping of current events

IV. Foundation or hidden aspect: what unconscious or hidden forces are at work in the situation (or perhaps you are working them!)

V.   Near future: what will happen as a result of past and present actions, energies, events and influences

VI. Past: the defining event or energy of the past that influenced and shaped present and future events

VII. Your influence: how your state of mind and approach are affecting the situation, for better or worse

VIII. Surrounding influences: how others' opinions, actions and approach are affecting the situation, for better or worse

IX. An unforeseen aspect: something or someone that affects or brings about the final outcome

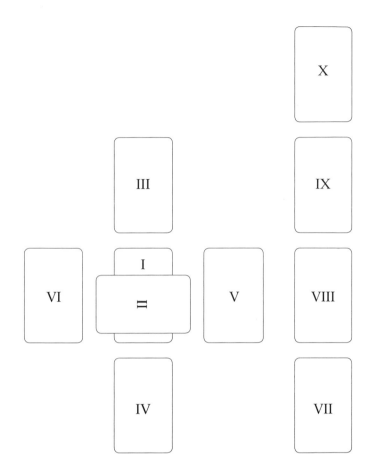

X. The final outcome or resolution: the concluding feeling, moment or event

Relationships Layout

Be it a personal, family or business relationship, this layout is designed specifically to help determine yours and another's feelings for each other, and how they might progress.

- When shuffling the cards, first hold the specific question in mind: 'How does "X" feel about me?'
- Then, without emotionally projecting what you think you already know, ask: 'How do I feel about "X"?'
- Then, lay two rows of five cards. The top row indicates how "X" feels about you and the bottom row how you feel about "X".

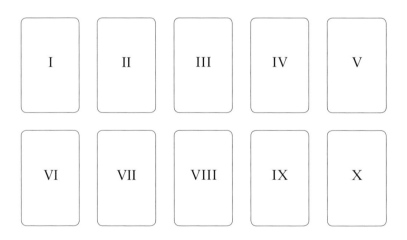

I.   How 'X' felt about you in the past: the defining event or energy of the past that subsequently influenced and shaped present and future events

II.   Past: another significant influence that helped shape the feelings of 'X' for you in the present moment

III.   Present: how 'X' feels about you right now, as a result of past influences, and what will happen in the future as a result, although sometimes efforts can be made to change the outcome

IV.   Hidden aspect: what hidden or unconscious forces are shaping how 'X' feels about you

V.   Near-future outcome: how 'X' will feel about you in the near future, as a result of past and present actions, energies, events and influences

VI.   How I felt about 'X' in the past: the defining event or energy of the past that subsequently influenced and shaped present and future events

VII. Past: another significant influence that helped shape my feelings for 'X' in the present moment

VIII. Present: how I feel about 'X' right now, as a result of past influences, and what will happen in the future as a result, although efforts can sometimes be made to change the outcome

IX.   Hidden aspect: what hidden or unconscious forces are shaping how I feel about 'X'

X.   Near-future outcome: how I will feel about 'X' in the near future, as a result of past and present actions, energies, events and influences

Future Extension Cards

If you want to know how the feelings of each individual will progress in the future, you can add extension cards to this reading by spreading the remaining deck of cards, picture face down, across the table and randomly selecting a few more cards – between three and five more per person. These cards should be read as an extension of the Near-Future Outcome card, except they represent the subsequent future possibilities as time progresses.